Clinical Updates on Perioperative Pain Management

Editors

Felice Eugenio Agro
Giuseppe Pascarella
Fabio Costa

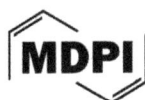 Basel • Beijing • Wuhan • Barcelona • Belgrade • Novi Sad • Cluj • Manchester

Editors

Felice Eugenio Agro
Fondazione Policlinico
Universitario Campus
Bio-Medico
Rome
Italy

Giuseppe Pascarella
Fondazione Policlinico
Universitario Campus
Bio-Medico
Rome
Italy

Fabio Costa
Fondazione Policlinico
Universitario Campus
Bio-Medico
Rome
Italy

Editorial Office
MDPI AG
Grosspeteranlage 5
4052 Basel, Switzerland

This is a reprint of articles from the Special Issue published online in the open access journal *Journal of Clinical Medicine* (ISSN 2077-0383) (available at: https://www.mdpi.com/journal/jcm/special_issues/F925ASF1UQ).

For citation purposes, cite each article independently as indicated on the article page online and as indicated below:

Lastname, A.A.; Lastname, B.B. Article Title. *Journal Name* **Year**, *Volume Number*, Page Range.

ISBN 978-3-7258-2215-7 (Hbk)
ISBN 978-3-7258-2216-4 (PDF)
doi.org/10.3390/books978-3-7258-2216-4

Contents

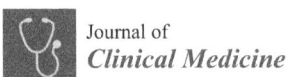

Review

The Analysis of Multiple Outcomes between General and Regional Anesthesia in Hip Fracture Surgery: A Systematic Review and Meta-Analysis of Randomized Controlled Trials

Dmitriy Viderman [1,*], Mina Aubakirova [1], Fatima Nabidollayeva [2] and Yerkin G. Abdildin [2]

[1] Department of Surgery, School of Medicine, Nazarbayev University, Astana 020000, Kazakhstan; mina.aubakirova@nu.edu.kz
[2] School of Engineering and Digital Sciences, Nazarbayev University, Astana 010000, Kazakhstan; fatima.nabidollayeva@nu.edu.kz (F.N.); yerkin.abdildin@nu.edu.kz (Y.G.A.)
* Correspondence: drviderman@gmail.com

Abstract: Surgical interventions in hip fracture have been associated with multiple adverse events, including perioperative hypotension and mortality, making the choice of the anesthetic method for this procedure crucial. There is still no consensus on whether regional (RA) or general (GA) anesthesia should be used to maintain hemodynamic stability and more favorable outcomes. Therefore, this meta-analysis examines the differences between RA and GA groups in the incidence of mortality, intraoperative hypotension, and other intra- and postoperative complications. The comparison is essential given the rising global prevalence of hip fractures and the need to optimize anesthesia strategies for improved patient outcomes, particularly in an aging population. We followed PRISMA guidelines (PROSPERO #CRD42022320413). We conducted the search for studies published in English before March 2022 in PubMed, Google Scholar, and the Cochrane Library. We included RCTs that compared general and regional anesthesia in adult patients having hip fracture surgical interventions. The primary outcome was perioperative mortality. The secondary outcomes were peri- or postoperative complications and duration of hospital stay. We conducted a meta-analysis in RevMan (version 5.4). We examined the quality of the methodology with the Cochrane risk of bias 2 tool, while the quality of evidence was determined with GRADE. Fifteen studies with 4110 patients were included. Our findings revealed no significant difference between general and regional anesthesia in risk of perioperative mortality (RR = 1.42 [0.96, 2.10], *p*-value = 0.08), intraoperative complications, or duration of hospital length of stay. Our results suggest that regional anesthesia and general anesthesia have comparable safety and can be used as alternatives based on specific patient requirements.

Keywords: general anesthesia; regional anesthesia; spinal anesthesia; epidural anesthesia; hip fracture; surgery; outcomes

Citation: Viderman, D.; Aubakirova, M.; Nabidollayeva, F.; Abdildin, Y.G. The Analysis of Multiple Outcomes between General and Regional Anesthesia in Hip Fracture Surgery: A Systematic Review and Meta-Analysis of Randomized Controlled Trials. *J. Clin. Med.* **2023**, *12*, 7513. https://doi.org/10.3390/jcm12247513

Academic Editor: Felice Eugenio Agro

Received: 19 October 2023
Revised: 21 November 2023
Accepted: 23 November 2023
Published: 5 December 2023

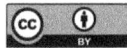

1. Introduction

The number of new cases of hip fracture is projected to exceed two and a half million worldwide by the first quarter of the 21st century [1]. Hip fracture is associated with a substantial perioperative complication rate of 6–19% overall [2,3] and a mortality rate of 3–8% [4–7]. Among complications, hypotension poses a particular concern, especially in the frail elderly population, given its association with elevated mortality at 30 days [8,9]. Different methods of anesthetic techniques, fluid therapy, and vasopressors are used to maintain the stability of the mean arterial pressure (MAP) [10,11]. Moreover, directing fluid and vasopressor administration based on a thorough hemodynamic evaluation, conducted through preoperative echocardiography and noninvasive monitoring, is crucial due to the potential adverse events associated with hypo- and hypervolemia. Hypovolemia may lead to decreased preload, resulting in cardiac output reduction and inadequate organ perfusion, while hypervolemia can cause systemic and pulmonary congestion, leading to decreased organ function. Currently, there are several approaches to monitoring fluid responsiveness. One option is the visualization of the inferior vena cava (IVC) diameter with echocardiography from the subcostal region or using a coronal trans-hepatic approach, although more research is needed to determine the appropriate thresholds for fluid responsiveness when employing the latter [12]. Alternatively, continuous noninvasive blood pressure monitoring can be used as it has been associated with a lower incidence of hypotension and hypertension during general anesthesia compared to intermittent cuff measurement [13]. Furthermore, the use of artificial intelligence for continuous noninvasive monitoring of blood pressure during general anesthesia has demonstrated promising results in hemodynamic assessment [14]. Despite the various attempts to prevent hypotensive events and other adverse outcomes, a definitive agreement on the best anesthesia approach for this surgery has not been reached.

General anesthesia (GA) is still widely used in hip fracture surgery, yet multiple regional anesthetic (RA) techniques are also gaining popularity. Thus, spinal anesthesia (SA) is often favored over general anesthesia in patients with a higher susceptibility to complications due to its effectiveness, simplicity, and minimal impact on cognitive and pulmonary function [15]. In fact, between 2007 and 2017, the usage of SA for hip fracture surgery increased by 50% [16]. However, SA is associated with severe hypotension, as it reduces the body's ability to compensate for changes in blood pressure, particularly in frail populations with numerous underlying health conditions [17]. On the other hand, continuous spinal anesthesia (CSA) has been shown to more effectively maintain hemodynamic stability compared with single-shot SA or GA thanks to low-fractionated administration of local anesthetic [10,11,18]. A recent meta-analysis also demonstrated that a 6.5 mg dose of SA was effective and associated with a lower incidence of hypotension compared to a 10.5 mg dose [19]. The authors suggest that a smaller dose provides an effective sensory block in conjunction with opiates through synergistic action of the two while minimizing systemic effects, including hemodynamic outcomes [19]. Similarly, multiple nerve blocks (MNBs) have been used as a GA alternative to minimize hypotensive episodes with some studies reporting promising results [20,21].

This systematic review with meta-analysis (SR&MA) aims to answer two main questions: Are there differences in death rates between the general and regional (SA, CSA, MNB) anesthesia groups? Are there differences in hypotension and other intraoperative and postoperative complications between the two groups?

2. Materials and Methods

2.1. Protocol

We conducted this study using the PRISMA guidelines [22]. PRISMA diagram is available in Figure 1. The protocol was developed prior to conducting the study and is publicly available in PROSPERO (#CRD42022320413). There were no deviations from the protocol.

2.2. Search Strategy and Criteria

The systematic search for relevant articles published before 15 March 2022 was performed using the following databases: PubMed, Google Scholar, and the Cochrane Library. The search terms used are available in Supplementary Materials. After searching the databases, a manual search was conducted by going through the references of the identified studies.

2.3. Screening

Screening of the articles was conducted by two authors in an independent manner. In case of disagreements, a third author was consulted. The studies were screened based on titles, then abstracts, and finally, by full texts. We included studies based on these criteria:

Inclusion criteria:

- Randomized controlled trials (RCTs);
- Adult patients with hip fractures undergoing surgical procedures;
- Comparing regional anesthesia versus general anesthesia;
- Reporting outcomes of interest: mortality (primary) and intra- and postoperative complications (secondary).

Exclusion criteria:

- Study designs other than RCTs;
- Pediatric studies;
- Not comparing regional to general anesthesia;
- Not reporting outcomes of interest.

Studies that did not meet the specified inclusion criteria were excluded.

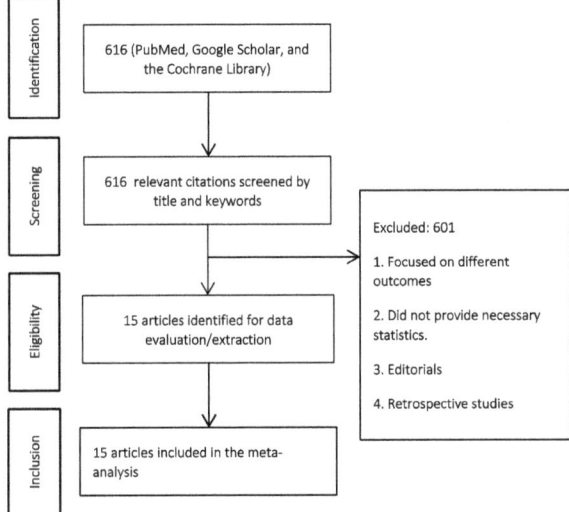

Figure 1. PRISMA diagram.

2.4. Data Extraction and Statistical Methods

Two authors extracted data independently. Any disagreements were solved by consulting a third author. We extracted study characteristics (country, primary/secondary outcomes, sample size, age) in a data table (Supplementary Table S1). Numeric data on the outcomes of interest were extracted into a spreadsheet for further analysis. If a study did not report data on an outcome of interest for this meta-analysis, we did not include that study in the analysis of that outcome. The primary outcome was death, while the secondary ones were other adverse events and duration of hospitalization. For each outcome, the risk ratio or standardized mean difference was calculated, and sensitivity analysis was conducted. If required, we employed mathematical techniques to calculate the sample mean and standard deviation [23,24]. Given the differences in study populations and procedures, a high level of heterogeneity among the studies was anticipated. Therefore, the random effects model was employed for the analysis. A significance level of $p < 0.05$ was adopted. Forest plots were constructed for each outcome. To assess statistical heterogeneity, we utilized the I^2 statistic. The data analysis was performed in the software "Review Manager (RevMan) [Computer program]. Version 5.4 (The Cochrane Collaboration, 2020, Copenhagen, Denmark)".

2.5. Quality Assessment

The quality of the methodology of the studies included in the review was evaluated with the Cochrane Risk of Bias Tool 2 [25]. We evaluated each study as "low risk", "some concerns", or "high risk" of bias based on the "randomization process", "deviations from the intended intervention", "missing outcome data", "measurement of the outcome", and "selection of the reported results". To assess the quality of the evidence of the main outcomes, we analyzed them with the GRADE [26]. We analyzed each outcome for "risk of bias", "inconsistency", "indirectness", and "imprecision" and summarized the overall quality of the outcome as "high", "moderate", "low", or "very low".

3. Results

3.1. Included Studies

The systematic search yielded 616 articles. After duplicate removal and title screening, 15 RCTs comprising 4110 patients were identified for inclusion in the MA [27–41] (Figure 1, Table 1).

Table 1. Characteristics of the included studies.

First Author, Year	Country	Groups	Study Outcomes	Age (Mean ± SD)	N of Patients: Total (I/C)	Local Anesthetic
Bigler, 1985 [27]	NG	GA SA	Prim.—postoperative mental function and morbidity	80.1 ± 1.6 77.6 ± 2.3	40 (20/20)	SA: 3 mL bupivacaine 0.75%
Davis, 1981 [28]	New Zealand	GA SA	Prim.—morbidity and mortality	81 ± 8.2 78 ± 8.6	132 (64/68)	SA: tetracaine 0.5% in 6% dextrose with adrenaline 1:100,000 without barbotage in 51 patients Hyperbaric cinchocaine 0.5% in 6% dextrose in 13 patients
Davis, 1987 [29]	New Zealand	GA SA	Prim.—mortality	79.5 ± 8.8	538 (259/279)	SA: tetracaine, nupercaine or bupivacaine (optional), hyper/iso-baric
Juelsgaard, 1998 [30]	Denmark	GA ISA SDSA	Prim.—incidence of myocardial ischemia in atherosclerotic patients	85.7 (72–94) 82.2 (65–99) 79.6 (72–92)	43 (14/15/14)	ISA: Bupivacaine 0.5% plain SDSA: 2.5 mL bupivacaine plain
Li, 2021 [31]	China	GA SA EA NB	Prim.—delirium within 7 days. Sec.—delirium characteristics, pain intensity in week 1, death at 30 days, hospital LoS, complications, and long-term and financial outcomes	77 (72–82) 77 (71–82)	942 (471/471)	SA: ropivacaine EA, NB: ropivacaine, bupivacaine, lidocaine
McKenzie, 1980 [32]	UK	GA SA	Prim.—postoperative arterial oxygenation and intraoperative mortality	76.8 ± 1.38 74.5 ± 2.29	100 (49/51)	SA: 1.3–1.5 mL hyperbaric cinchocaine 0.5%
McKenzie, 1984 [33]	UK	GA SA	Prim.—mortality at 1 year	74.2 ± 1.7 75.4 ± 1.4	150 (75/75)	SA: 1.3–1.5 mL hyperbaric 0.5% cinchocaine
McKenzie, 1985 [34]	UK	GA SA	Prim.—incidence of deep vein thrombosis and pulmonary embolism	73.9 ± 4.1 72.3 ± 2.8	40 (20/20)	SA: 1.2–1.5 mL hyperbaric conchocaine
McLaren, 1978 [35]	UK	GA SA	Prim.—mortality and morbidity	76 ± 9.7 75.6 ± 10.3	55 (26/29)	SA: 0.5 mL hyperbaric cinchocaine (0.5% in 6% dextrose)
Messina, 2013 [36]	Italy	GA SA	Prim.—hemodynamic response	81.8 ± 6.3 83.9 ± 9.4	20 (10/10)	SA: 7.5 mg levobupivacaine diluted from 7.5 mg/mL with 2 mL distilled water + preservative-free sufentanil 5 μg
Neuman, 2021 [37]	USA, Canada	GA SA	Prim—death or inability to walk independently at 60 days after randomization	77.7 ± 10.7 78.4 ± 10.6	1572 (782/790)	Varied across study sites
Parker, 2015 [38]	UK	GA SA	Prim.—mortality	82.9 (range 52–105) 83.0 (range 59–99)	322 (158/164)	At the discretion of the anesthetist
Svartling, 1986 [39]	Finland	GA SA	Prim.—arterial blood, pressure, arterial oxygen tension, plasma levels of cortisol	79.6 ± 2.1 75.1 ± 1.1	30 (15/15)	SA: 3 mL isobaric bupivacaine hydrochloride 0.5%
Tzimas, 2018 [40]	Greece	GA SA	Prim.—POCD at 30 days after surgery, possible differences Sec.—delirium on days 1, 2, 3, 4	77.11 ± 6.5 75.09 ± 6.08	70 (37/33)	SA: fentanyl 20 mcg + ropivacaine 0.75% based on somatometric characteristics
White, 1980 [41]	South Africa	GA SA PCB	Prim.—pre, intra-, and postoperative events and mortality	78 ± 7.8 80 ± 9.1 78 ± 7.3	56 (20/20/16)	SA: hyperbaric cinchocaine 0.6–0.8 mL

Abbreviations: C, control; I, intervention; N, number; POCD, postoperative cognitive dysfunction; prim., primary outcome; sec., secondary outcome; SD, standard deviation; GA, general anesthesia; SA, spinal anesthesia; ISA, incremental spinal anesthesia; SDSA, single-dose spinal anesthesia; PCB, psoas compartment block; EA, epidural block; NB, nerve blocks; NG, not given; LoS, length of stay.

3.2. Mortality

There was no difference in the risk of death in the RA group compared to the GA group (RR = 1.42; 95% CI: [0.96, 2.10], *p*-value = 0.08) (Figure 2). Sensitivity analysis revealed that excluding either Davis et al. (1987) [29] or Li et al. (2022) [31] changed the result favoring RA. We should note that most included studies reported values for the period of four weeks or one month, Neuman et al. (2021) [37] reported values for the period of "after 60 days", and Bigler et al. (1985) [27] did not mention the specific postoperative period.

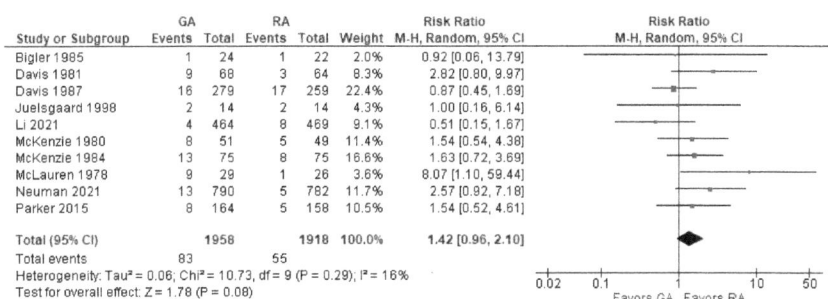

Figure 2. Death. Square—risk ratio for individual studies; line—confidence interval; diamond—pooled risk ratio [27–33,37,38].

3.3. Intraoperative Hypotension

We did not observe a difference between the RA and the GA groups in the risk of hypotension (RR = 1.24 [0.59, 2.60], *p* = 0.57) (Figure 3). Among the six studies with 1095 patients, there was substantial heterogeneity at I^2 = 76%.

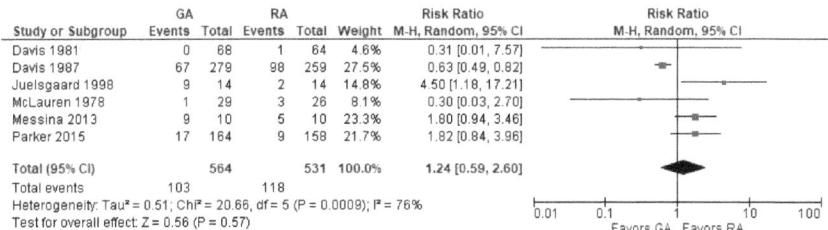

Figure 3. Intraoperative hypotension. Square—risk ratio for individual studies; line—confidence interval; diamond—pooled risk ratio [28–30,35,36,38].

3.4. Cardiac and Cerebrovascular Complications

We combined myocardial infarction, cardiac failure, and cardiovascular accident into the overall cardiac and cerebrovascular complications outcome. There was no significant difference between the GA and RA groups in terms of myocardial infarction (RR = 1.23 [0.54, 2.82]), cardiac failure (RR = 0.85 [0.23, 3.07]), or cerebrovascular accident (RR = 0.60 [0.03, 12.83]). The lack of difference was maintained at the exclusion of any study (Figure 4).

3.5. Vascular Complications

For deep vein thrombosis, there was no difference between the two groups at RR = 1.36 [0.43, 4.29]. It should be mentioned that the result changed in favor of RA when the study by McKenzie et al. (1985) [34] was excluded. For postoperative pulmonary embolus, the results for the two groups were comparable at RR = 1.59 [0.61, 4.14] (Figure 5). The overall result of the model for vascular complications is in favor of RA.

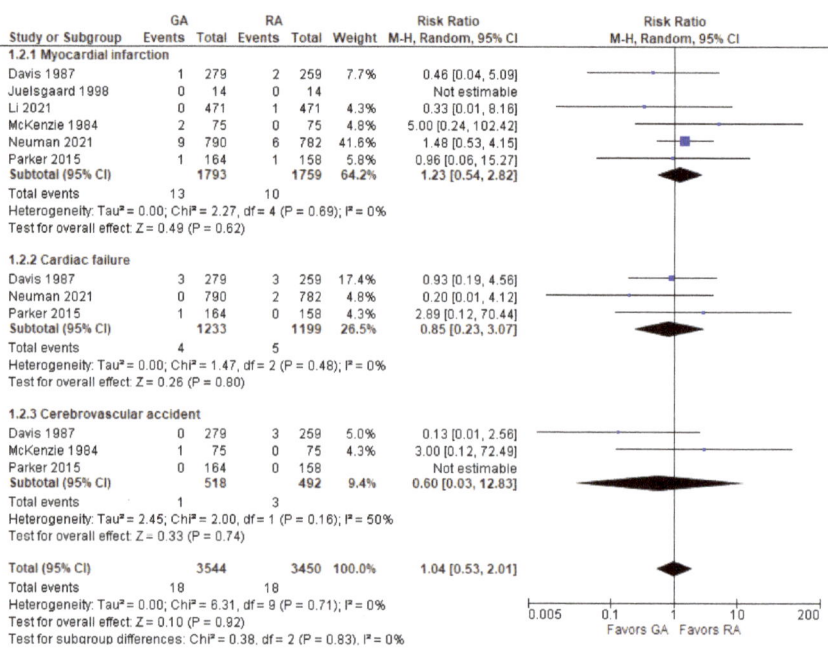

Figure 4. Cardiac and cerebrovascular complications. Square—risk ratio for individual studies; line—confidence interval; diamond—pooled risk ratio [29–31,33,37,38].

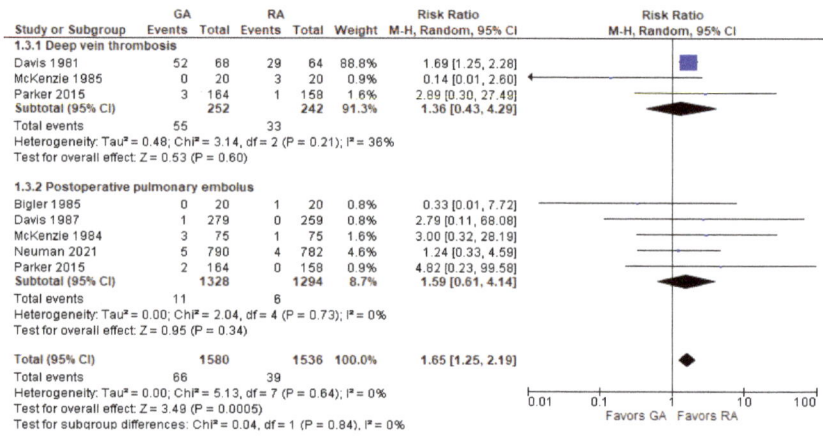

Figure 5. Vascular complications. Square—risk ratio for individual studies; line—confidence interval; diamond—pooled risk ratio [27–29,33,34,37,38].

3.6. Acute Kidney Disease

The model does not favor RA over GA (Figure 6) since RR with 95% CI is equal to 1.68 [0.28, 10.27].

3.7. Postoperative Pneumonia

The model does not favor RA over GA (Figure 7) since RR with 95% CI is equal to 1.19 [0.73, 1.96].

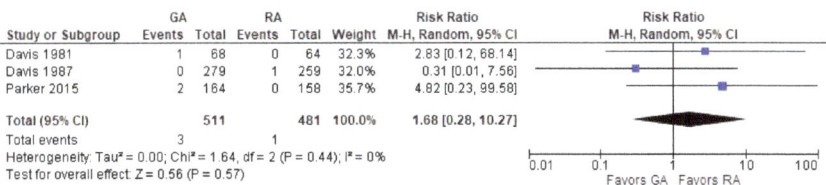

Figure 6. Acute kidney disease. Square—risk ratio for individual studies; line—confidence interval; diamond—pooled risk ratio [28,29,38].

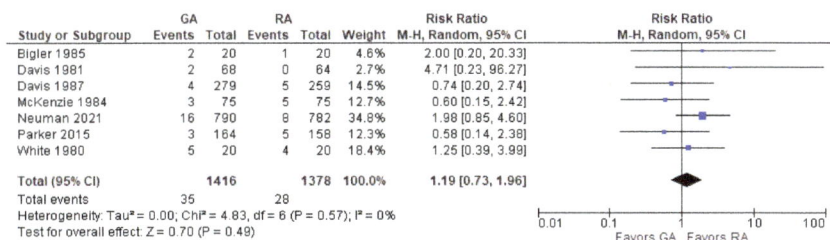

Figure 7. Postoperative pneumonia. Square—risk ratio for individual studies; line—confidence interval; diamond—pooled risk ratio [27–29,33,37,38,41].

3.8. Intraoperative Blood Loss (mL)

The model does not favor RA over GA (Figure 8) since the std. mean difference (SMD) with 95% CI is equal to 0.24 [−1.34, 1.83].

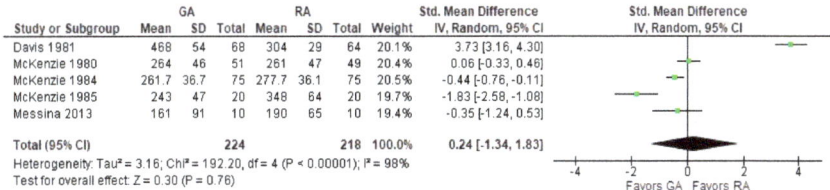

Figure 8. Intraoperative blood loss (mL). Square—risk ratio for individual studies; line—confidence interval; diamond—pooled risk ratio [28,32–34,36].

3.9. Perioperative Blood Transfusion

The model (Figure 9) does not favor RA over GA since RR with 95% CI is equal to 1.04 [0.96, 1.13].

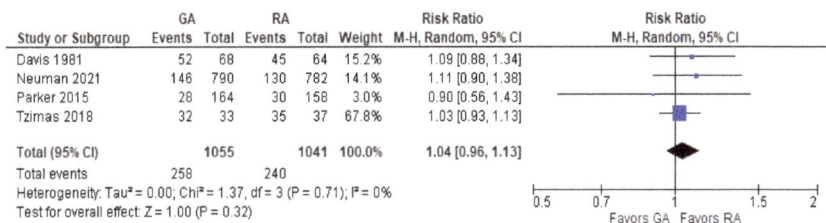

Figure 9. Perioperative blood transfusion. Square—risk ratio for individual studies; line—confidence interval; diamond—pooled risk ratio [27,37,38,40].

3.10. Duration of Hospital Stay (Days)

The model does not favor RA over GA (Figure 10) since SMD with 95% CI is equal to 0.33 [−0.08, 0.74].

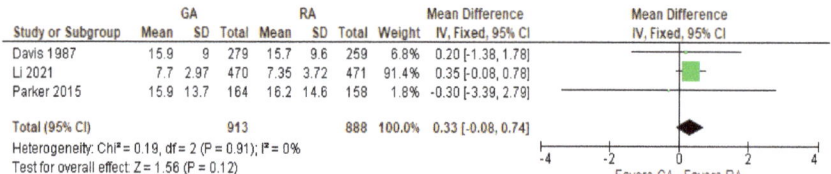

Figure 10. Duration of hospital stay (days). Green square—risk ratio for individual studies; line—confidence interval; diamond—pooled risk ratio [29,31,38].

3.11. Quality Assessment

We report the Cochrane Risk of Bias 2 in Table 2. Given the nature of the intervention, group assignment could not be concealed from the patients, which contributed to the "risk of bias". Moreover, the randomization process and concealment technique were not described in the older publications. However, these were published in reputable journals. Therefore, all the studies were rated as having "some concerns" in terms of risk of bias.

Table 2. Cochrane risk of bias.

Study (Author, Year)	Risk of Bias Arising from the Randomization Process	Risk of Bias Due to Deviations from the Intended Interventions	Missing Outcome Data	Risk of Bias in Measurement of the Outcome	Risk of Bias in Selection of the Reported Result	Overall Risk of Bias
Davis et al., 1981 [28]	Some concerns	Low risk	Low risk	Some concerns	Low risk	Some concerns
Bigler et al., 1985 [27]	Some concerns	Low risk	Low risk	Some concerns	Low risk	Some concerns
Davis et al., 1987 [29]	Some concerns	Low risk	Low risk	Some concerns	Low risk	Some concerns
Juelsgaard et al., 1998 [30]	Some concerns	Low risk	Low risk	Some concerns	Low risk	Some concerns
Mckenzie et al., 1980 [32]	Some concerns	Low risk	Low risk	Some concerns	Low risk	Some concerns
Mckenzie et al., 1984 [33]	Some concerns	Low risk	Low risk	Some concerns	Low risk	Some concerns
Neuman et al., 2021 [37]	Low risk	Low risk	Some concerns	Some concerns	Low risk	Some concerns
Parker et al., 2015 [38]	Low risk	Some concerns	Low risk	Low risk	Low risk	Some concerns
White et al., 1980 [41]	Some concerns	Low risk	Low risk	Some concerns	Low risk	Some concerns
Messina et al., 2013 [36]	Low risk	Low risk	Low risk	Some concerns	Low risk	Some concerns
Svartling et al., 1986 [39]	Some concerns	Low risk	Low risk	Some concerns	Low risk	Some concerns
McLaren et al., 1978 [35]	Some concerns	Low risk	Low risk	Some concerns	Low risk	Some concerns
Li et al., 2022 [31]	Low risk	Low risk	Low risk	Some concerns	Low risk	Some concerns
Tzimas et al., 2018 [40]	Some concerns	Low risk	Low risk	Some concerns	Low risk	Some concerns
McKenzie et al., 1985 [34]	Some concerns	Low risk	Low risk	Some concerns	Low risk	Some concerns

The results of the GRADE assessment of the main outcomes are presented in Table 3. The outcomes ranged in the quality of evidence from "low" to "very low" due to "risk of bias" (lack of blinding, lack of information concerning allocation concealment, etc.), "inconsistency" (unexplained heterogeneity and wide variance of point estimates), and "imprecision" (wide confidence intervals). The full description of the assessment is available in the Evidence profile (Table S1).

Table 3. Summary of findings. Abbreviations: CI, confidence interval; GA, general anesthesia; GRADE, Grading of Recommendations Assessment, Development and Evaluation; N, number; RA, regional anesthesia; RCT, randomized controlled trial.

Outcome	N of Studies	Design	N of Patients RA	N of Patients GA	Effect Relative Risk/Mean Difference [95% CI]	Overall Quality
Death	10	RCT	1918	1958	1.42 [0.96, 2.10]	Low [a] ⊕⊕⊖⊖
Intraoperative hypotension	6	RCT	564	531	1.24 [0.59, 2.60]	Low [a] ⊕⊕⊖⊖
Myocardial infarction	6	RCT	1759	1793	1.23 [0.54, 2.82]	Very low [b] ⊕⊖⊖⊖
Cardiac failure	3	RCT	1199	1233	0.85 [0.23, 3.07]	Very low [b] ⊕⊖⊖⊖
Cerebrovascular accident	3	RCT	492	518	0.60 [0.03, 12.83]	Very low [b] ⊕⊖⊖⊖
Deep vein thrombosis	3	RCT	252	242	1.36 [0.43, 4.29]	Very low [b] ⊕⊖⊖⊖
Postoperative pulmonary embolus	5	RCT	1294	1328	1.59 [0.61, 4.14]	Very low [b] ⊕⊖⊖⊖

[a] Due to the risk of bias and inconsistency. [b] Due to the risk of bias, inconsistency, and imprecision. ⊕⊕⊖⊖—low quality; ⊕⊖⊖⊖—very low quality.

4. Discussion

There are controversies as to the most appropriate anesthetic approach in hip fracture surgeries to minimize the risk of complications, especially among the frail population. In this meta-analysis, we failed to identify the benefits of RA or GA for hip fracture surgery concerning mortality as well as intra- and postoperative complications.

The primary outcome was death. Although there was a trend toward decreased risk of mortality in the RA group at RR = 1.42 [0.96, 2.10], *p*-value = 0.08, we failed to reach statistical significance. Therefore, we observed no difference between the groups. On the contrary, previous observational studies concluded that GA might have an association with reduced incidence of mortality, adverse events, delirium, and shorter length of hospital stay compared with SA [42–46].

The secondary outcomes were intra- and postoperative complications. The results between the two groups were comparable. This finding is in agreement with a recent study that found no difference between the CSA/MNB and GA groups concerning postoperative complications and mortality rates in elderly patients undergoing hip fracture surgery [47]. However, in their study, CSA and MNB offered superior intraoperative blood pressure (BP) control than GA and comparable BP control between the regional anesthesia groups. Moreover, the MNB and CSA groups had a decreased frequency of cases of hypotension below 50 mmHg and requirement in vasopressors compared with the GA group.

One of the reasons for discrepancies in our results with previous literature might be the variations in the characteristics of the patient populations across studies, such as differences in age distribution, baseline health conditions, or comorbidities. These factors may interact differently with the chosen anesthesia methods, influencing mortality and other intra- and postoperative outcomes. Additionally, variations in surgical and anesthetic protocols, including drug dosages, administration techniques, and perioperative care, could contribute to differing results. Methodological dissimilarities, such as study design and blinding procedures, might also play a role in the observed differences. The evolution of medical practices over the study period, spanning three decades, could introduce disparities in outcomes due to advancements in surgical and anesthetic techniques.

Thus, our results suggest that the rate of death and adverse events in patients undergoing surgical procedures for hip fracture did not differ significantly between GA and

RA, suggesting comparable safety of the two approaches. This might suggest that either approach can be used as an alternative based on specific patient requirements. For example, RA may be favored in patients with cardiovascular or pulmonary comorbidities, as it can offer better hemodynamic stability. RA was hypothesized to have minimal impact on cognitive function, making it a preferred option for elderly patients. However, a recent meta-analysis did not support this hypothesis [48]. Certain regional techniques, like Continuous Spinal Anesthesia or Multiple Nerve Blocks, may provide superior intraoperative blood pressure control compared to GA. On the other hand, patients with contraindications to regional techniques, such as severe coagulopathy or hemodynamic instability, may be more suitable for general anesthesia. GA might also be preferred in emergency cases or when a rapid onset of anesthesia is crucial. A recent study also proposed that the decision on the anesthesia type for hip fracture surgery may be influenced more by patient preference rather than solely relying on existing evidence and variations in clinical results [46]. For instance, some patients may prefer GA due to a desire for complete unconsciousness during the procedure. Ultimately, the choice between GA and RA should be made on a case-by-case basis, taking into account the patient's medical history, preferences, and the specific clinical context. Shared decision-making between the patient and the healthcare team is crucial to ensure the most appropriate and individualized anesthesia approach for hip fracture surgery.

Thus, the comparable efficacy of GA and RA in hip fracture surgery has substantial implications for clinical decision-making. This finding supports a personalized approach to anesthesia selection, enabling clinicians to consider individual patient characteristics, such as cardiovascular and pulmonary comorbidities or the risk of postoperative cognitive dysfunction. Moreover, the study suggests considering patient preferences in anesthesia choice, promoting shared decision-making processes. Additionally, the study's results suggest that in cases with contraindications to spinal anesthesia, GA remains a viable and safe option. Overall, the study's insights enhance the practical relevance of clinical decision-making by providing a nuanced understanding of when and how to apply GA and RA based on individual patient needs and preferences.

There are several limitations in the body of evidence. The majority of the included studies were conducted over three decades ago, potentially misaligning with current standards in surgical and anesthetic practices. Moreover, the studies demonstrated significant methodological limitations, including a lack of blinding and an inadequate description of the randomization method, which may introduce bias. The review process itself had limitations, as it combined studies with variations in anesthetic regimens and blocks, and there were relative differences in patients' conditions at admission, with some studies defining outcomes differently. Additionally, the inclusion of studies spanning over 40 years may have introduced variations in the quality and safety of surgical and anesthetic techniques. These limitations suggest that generalizing the findings to contemporary clinical settings should be carried out with caution. Moreover, a methodological limitation of our study is the absence of trial sequential analysis (TSA) to assess the robustness of our meta-analysis findings. TSA is an increasingly utilized statistical method in medical literature designed to manage type I and type II errors in meta-analyses [49,50]. It involves cumulative analysis, adjusting significance thresholds, and statistical power throughout the process.

Considering that the majority of the included studies were conducted over three decades ago, future research should involve RCTs that align with current clinical standards. Researchers should also pay careful attention to issues such as blinding and provide detailed descriptions of the randomization method to enhance the quality and reliability of study outcomes. Standardized reporting of outcomes and procedures across studies would facilitate meaningful comparisons and meta-analyses. Long-term outcomes, especially in terms of recovery trajectories, should be investigated to understand the overall impact of anesthesia choice on patient recovery. Patient preferences in anesthesia decision-making are also an issue that should be explored. Addressing these aspects in future research will contribute to a more comprehensive and clinically relevant understanding of the choice between general and regional anesthesia in hip fracture surgeries. Future meta-analyses could perform a subgroup analysis based on the years of publication to partially solve the issue of including older studies.

The comparable safety and efficacy of general and regional anesthesia observed in our meta-analysis suggest that either approach can be acceptable, depending on individual patient characteristics, preferences, and clinical contexts. Policymakers and guideline developers may find it valuable to acknowledge this flexibility and consider incorporating it into recommendations. This recognition can provide healthcare practitioners with a broader choice of options and encourage shared decision-making between patients and clinicians. Additionally, our study highlights the importance of ongoing updates to clinical guidelines to reflect contemporary evidence and advancements in anesthesia techniques.

5. Conclusions

Existing evidence showed that the rate of mortality in patients undergoing hip fracture surgery did not differ significantly between general anesthesia and regional anesthesia. There was no statistically significant difference between RA and GA in cardiac and cerebral complications, including myocardial infarction, cardiac failure, cerebrovascular accident, deep vein thrombosis, postoperative pulmonary embolus, renal failure, postoperative pneumonia, intraoperative hypotension, intraoperative blood loss, intraoperative blood transfusion, or duration of hospital length of stay.

Supplementary Materials: The following supporting information can be downloaded at https://www.mdpi.com/article/10.3390/jcm12247513/s1, Document S1: Search terms; Table S1: Evidence profile.

Author Contributions: Conceptualization, D.V.; methodology, D.V.; data extraction, M.A.; software, Y.G.A. and F.N.; formal analysis, Y.G.A. and F.N.; quality assessment, M.A.; writing—original draft preparation, D.V.; writing—review and editing, D.V., M.A., F.N. and Y.G.A. All authors have read and agreed to the published version of the manuscript.

Funding: This work was supported in part by Nazarbayev University Faculty Development Competitive Research Grants No. SOM2021005 (021220FD2851) and 11022021FD2906. The authors have no other relevant affiliations or financial involvement with any organization or entity with a financial interest in or financial conflict with the subject matter or materials discussed in the manuscript apart from those disclosed.

Institutional Review Board Statement: Not applicable.

Informed Consent Statement: Not applicable.

Data Availability Statement: No new data were created or analyzed in this study. Data sharing is not applicable to this article.

Conflicts of Interest: The authors declare no conflict of interest.

References

1. Gullberg, B.; Johnell, O.; Kanis, J.A. World-Wide Projections for Hip Fracture. *Osteoporos. Int.* **1997**, *7*, 407–413. [CrossRef] [PubMed]
2. Haugan, K.; Johnsen, L.G.; Basso, T.; Foss, O.A. Mortality and Readmission Following Hip Fracture Surgery: A Retrospective Study Comparing Conventional and Fast-Track Care. *BMJ Open* **2017**, *7*, e015574. [CrossRef] [PubMed]
3. White, S.M.; Griffiths, R. Projected Incidence of Proximal Femoral Fracture in England: A Report from the NHS Hip Fracture Anaesthesia Network (HIPFAN). *Injury* **2011**, *42*, 1230–1233. [CrossRef] [PubMed]
4. Johansen, A.; Tsang, C.; Boulton, C.; Wakeman, R.; Moppett, I. Understanding Mortality Rates after Hip Fracture Repair Using ASA Physical Status in the National Hip Fracture Database. *Anaesthesia* **2017**, *72*, 961–966. [CrossRef] [PubMed]
5. White, S.M.; Moppett, I.K.; Griffiths, R.; Johansen, A.; Wakeman, R.; Boulton, C.; Plant, F.; Williams, A.; Pappenheim, K.; Majeed, A.; et al. Secondary Analysis of Outcomes after 11,085 Hip Fracture Operations from the Prospective UK Anaesthesia Sprint Audit of Practice (ASAP-2). *Anaesthesia* **2016**, *71*, 506–514. [CrossRef] [PubMed]
6. Le Manach, Y.; Collins, G.; Bhandari, M.; Bessissow, A.; Boddaert, J.; Khiami, F.; Chaudhry, H.; De Beer, J.; Riou, B.; Landais, P.; et al. Outcomes After Hip Fracture Surgery Compared with Elective Total Hip Replacement. *JAMA* **2015**, *314*, 1159. [CrossRef]
7. Haentjens, P. Meta-Analysis: Excess Mortality After Hip Fracture Among Older Women and Men. *Ann. Intern. Med.* **2010**, *152*, 380. [CrossRef]

8. White, S.M.; Griffiths, R. Problems Defining 'Hypotension' in Hip Fracture Anaesthesia. *Br. J. Anaesth.* **2019**, *123*, e528–e529. [CrossRef]
9. Wesselink, E.M.; Kappen, T.H.; Torn, H.M.; Slooter, A.J.C.; Van Klei, W.A. Intraoperative Hypotension and the Risk of Postoperative Adverse Outcomes: A Systematic Review. *Br. J. Anaesth.* **2018**, *121*, 706–721. [CrossRef]
10. Biboulet, P.; Jourdan, A.; Van Haevre, V.; Morau, D.; Bernard, N.; Bringuier, S.; Capdevila, X. Hemodynamic Profile of Target-Controlled Spinal Anesthesia Compared with 2 Target-Controlled General Anesthesia Techniques in Elderly Patients with Cardiac Comorbidities. *Reg. Anesth. Pain Med.* **2012**, *37*, 433–440. [CrossRef]
11. Futier, E.; Lefrant, J.-Y.; Guinot, P.-G.; Godet, T.; Lorne, E.; Cuvillon, P.; Bertran, S.; Leone, M.; Pastene, B.; Piriou, V.; et al. Effect of Individualized vs Standard Blood Pressure Management Strategies on Postoperative Organ Dysfunction Among High-Risk Patients Undergoing Major Surgery: A Randomized Clinical Trial. *JAMA* **2017**, *318*, 1346. [CrossRef] [PubMed]
12. La Via, L.; Astuto, M.; Dezio, V.; Muscarà, L.; Palella, S.; Zawadka, M.; Vignon, P.; Sanfilippo, F. Agreement between Subcostal and Transhepatic Longitudinal Imaging of the Inferior Vena Cava for the Evaluation of Fluid Responsiveness: A Systematic Review. *J. Crit. Care* **2022**, *71*, 154108. [CrossRef] [PubMed]
13. Sanfilippo, F.; La Via, L.; Dezio, V.; Santonocito, C.; Amelio, P.; Genoese, G.; Astuto, M.; Noto, A. Assessment of the Inferior Vena Cava Collapsibility from Subcostal and Trans-Hepatic Imaging Using Both M-Mode or Artificial Intelligence: A Prospective Study on Healthy Volunteers. *Intensive Care Med. Exp.* **2023**, *11*, 15. [CrossRef] [PubMed]
14. Juri, T.; Suehiro, K.; Kimura, A.; Mukai, A.; Tanaka, K.; Yamada, T.; Mori, T.; Nishikawa, K. Impact of Continuous Non-Invasive Blood Pressure Monitoring on Hemodynamic Fluctuation during General Anesthesia: A Randomized Controlled Study. *J. Clin. Monit. Comput.* **2018**, *32*, 1005–1013. [CrossRef] [PubMed]
15. White, S.M.; Moppett, I.K.; Griffiths, R. Outcome by Mode of Anaesthesia for Hip Fracture Surgery. An Observational Audit of 65 535 Patients in a National Dataset. *Anaesthesia* **2014**, *69*, 224–230. [CrossRef] [PubMed]
16. Maxwell, B.G.; Spitz, W.; Porter, J. Association of Increasing Use of Spinal Anesthesia in Hip Fracture Repair with Treating an Aging Patient Population. *JAMA Surg.* **2020**, *155*, 167. [CrossRef]
17. Boddaert, J.; Raux, M.; Khiami, F.; Riou, B. Perioperative Management of Elderly Patients with Hip Fracture. *Anesthesiology* **2014**, *121*, 1336–1341. [CrossRef]
18. O'Donnell, C.M.; Black, N.; McCourt, K.C.; McBrien, M.E.; Clarke, M.; Patterson, C.C.; Blackwood, B.; McAuley, D.F.; Shields, M.O. Development of a Core Outcome Set for Studies Evaluating the Effects of Anaesthesia on Perioperative Morbidity and Mortality Following Hip Fracture Surgery. *Br. J. Anaesth.* **2019**, *122*, 120–130. [CrossRef]
19. Messina, A.; La Via, L.; Milani, A.; Savi, M.; Calabrò, L.; Sanfilippo, F.; Negri, K.; Castellani, G.; Cammarota, G.; Robba, C.; et al. Spinal Anesthesia and Hypotensive Events in Hip Fracture Surgical Repair in Elderly Patients: A Meta-Analysis. *J. Anesth. Analg. Crit. Care* **2022**, *2*, 19. [CrossRef]
20. Devisme, V.; Picart, F.; Lejouan, R.; Legrand, A.; Savry, C.; Morin, V. Combined Lumbar and Sacral Plexus Block Compared with Plain Bupivacaine Spinal Anesthesia for Hip Fractures in the Elderly. *Reg. Anesth. Pain Med.* **2000**, *25*, 158–162. [CrossRef]
21. Johnston, D.F.; Stafford, M.; McKinney, M.; Deyermond, R.; Dane, K. Peripheral Nerve Blocks with Sedation Using Propofol and Alfentanil Target-Controlled Infusion for Hip Fracture Surgery: A Review of 6 Years in Use. *J. Clin. Anesth.* **2016**, *29*, 33–39. [CrossRef]
22. Page, M.J.; McKenzie, J.E.; Bossuyt, P.M.; Boutron, I.; Hoffmann, T.C.; Mulrow, C.D.; Shamseer, L.; Tetzlaff, J.M.; Akl, E.A.; Brennan, S.E.; et al. The PRISMA 2020 Statement: An Updated Guideline for Reporting Systematic Reviews. *BMJ* **2021**, *372*, n71. [CrossRef] [PubMed]
23. Luo, D.; Wan, X.; Liu, J.; Tong, T. Optimally Estimating the Sample Mean from the Sample Size, Median, Mid-Range, and/or Mid-Quartile Range. *Stat. Methods Med. Res.* **2018**, *27*, 1785–1805. [CrossRef] [PubMed]
24. Wan, X.; Wang, W.; Liu, J.; Tong, T. Estimating the Sample Mean and Standard Deviation from the Sample Size, Median, Range and/or Interquartile Range. *BMC Med. Res. Methodol.* **2014**, *14*, 135. [CrossRef] [PubMed]
25. Sterne, J.A.C.; Savović, J.; Page, M.J.; Elbers, R.G.; Blencowe, N.S.; Boutron, I.; Cates, C.J.; Cheng, H.-Y.; Corbett, M.S.; Eldridge, S.M.; et al. RoB 2: A Revised Tool for Assessing Risk of Bias in Randomised Trials. *BMJ* **2019**, *366*, l4898. [CrossRef] [PubMed]
26. Guyatt, G.H.; Oxman, A.D.; Schünemann, H.J.; Tugwell, P.; Knottnerus, A. GRADE Guidelines: A New Series of Articles in the Journal of Clinical Epidemiology. *J. Clin. Epidemiol.* **2011**, *64*, 380–382. [CrossRef] [PubMed]
27. Bigler, D.; Adelhøj, B.; Petring, O.U.; Pederson, N.O.; Busch, P.; Kalhke, P. Mental Function and Morbidity after Acute Hip Surgery during Spinal and General Anaesthesia. *Anaesthesia* **1985**, *40*, 672–676. [CrossRef]
28. Davis, F.M.; Laurenson, V.G. Spinal Anaesthesia or General Anaesthesia for Emergency Hip Surgery in Elderly Patients. *Anaesth. Intensive Care* **1981**, *9*, 352–358. [CrossRef]
29. Davis, F.M.; Woolner, D.F.; Frampton, C.; Wilkinson, A.; Grant, A.; Harrison, R.T.; Roberts, M.T.S.; Thadaka, R. Prospective, Multi-Centre Trial of Mortality Following General or Spinal Anaesthesia for Hip Fracture Surgery in the Elderly. *Br. J. Anaesth.* **1987**, *59*, 1080–1088. [CrossRef]
30. Juelsgaard, P.; Sand, N.P.R.; Felsby, S.; Dalsgaard, J.; Jakobsen, K.B.; Brink, O.; Carlsson, P.S.; Thygesen, K. Perioperative Myocardial Ischaemia in Patients Undergoing Surgery for Fractured Hip Randomized to Incremental Spinal, Single-Dose Spinal or General Anaesthesia. *Eur. J. Anaesthesiol.* **1998**, *15*, 656–663. [CrossRef]

31. Li, T.; Li, J.; Yuan, L.; Wu, J.; Jiang, C.; Daniels, J.; Mehta, R.L.; Wang, M.; Yeung, J.; Jackson, T.; et al. Effect of Regional vs General Anesthesia on Incidence of Postoperative Delirium in Older Patients Undergoing Hip Fracture Surgery: The RAGA Randomized Trial. *JAMA* **2022**, *327*, 50. [CrossRef] [PubMed]
32. Mckenzie, P.J.; Wishart, H.Y.; Dewar, K.M.S.; Gray, I.; Smith, G. Comparison of the Effects of Spinal Anaesthesia and General Anaesthesia on Postoperative Oxygenation and Perioperative Mortality. *Br. J. Anaesth.* **1980**, *52*, 49–54. [CrossRef]
33. Mckenzie, P.J.; Wishart, H.Y.; Smith, G. Long-Term Outcome after Repair of Fractured Neck of Femur. *Br. J. Anaesth.* **1984**, *56*, 581–585. [CrossRef] [PubMed]
34. McKenzie, P.J.; Wishart, H.Y.; Gray, I.; Smith, G. Effects of Anaesthetic Technique on Deep Vein Thrombosis. *Br. J. Anaesth.* **1985**, *57*, 853–857. [CrossRef]
35. McLAREN, A.D.; Stockwell, M.C.; Reid, V.T. Anaesthetic Techniques for Surgical Correction of Fractured Neck of Femur.: A Comparative Study of Spinal and General Anaesthesia in the Elderly. *Anaesthesia* **1978**, *33*, 10–14. [CrossRef]
36. Messina, A.; Frassanito, L.; Colombo, D.; Vergari, A.; Draisci, G.; Della Corte, F.; Antonelli, M. Hemodynamic Changes Associated with Spinal and General Anesthesia for Hip Fracture Surgery in Severe ASA III Elderly Population: A Pilot Trial. *Minerva Anestesiol.* **2013**, *79*, 1021–1029. [PubMed]
37. Neuman, M.D.; Feng, R.; Carson, J.L.; Gaskins, L.J.; Dillane, D.; Sessler, D.I.; Sieber, F.; Magaziner, J.; Marcantonio, E.R.; Mehta, S.; et al. Spinal Anesthesia or General Anesthesia for Hip Surgery in Older Adults. *N. Engl. J. Med.* **2021**, *385*, 2025–2035. [CrossRef] [PubMed]
38. Parker, M.J.; Griffiths, R. General versus Regional Anaesthesia for Hip Fractures. A Pilot Randomised Controlled Trial of 322 Patients. *Injury* **2015**, *46*, 1562–1566. [CrossRef]
39. Svartling, N.; Lehtinen, A.-M.; Tarkkanen, L. The Effect of Anaesthesia on Changes in Blood Pressure and Plasma Cortisol Levels Induced by Cementation with Methylmethacrylate. *Acta Anaesthesiol. Scand.* **1986**, *30*, 247–252. [CrossRef]
40. Tzimas, P.; Samara, E.; Petrou, A.; Korompilias, A.; Chalkias, A.; Papadopoulos, G. The Influence of Anesthetic Techniques on Postoperative Cognitive Function in Elderly Patients Undergoing Hip Fracture Surgery: General vs Spinal Anesthesia. *Injury* **2018**, *49*, 2221–2226. [CrossRef]
41. White, I.W.C.; Chappell, W.A. Anaesthesia for Surgical Correction of Fractured Femoral Neck A Comparison of Three Techniques. *Anaesthesia* **1980**, *35*, 1107–1110. [CrossRef] [PubMed]
42. Neuman, M.D.; Silber, J.H.; Elkassabany, N.M.; Ludwig, J.M.; Fleisher, L.A. Comparative Effectiveness of Regional *versus* General Anesthesia for Hip Fracture Surgery in Adults. *Anesthesiology* **2012**, *117*, 72–92. [CrossRef] [PubMed]
43. Ahn, E.J.; Kim, H.J.; Kim, K.W.; Choi, H.R.; Kang, H.; Bang, S.R. Comparison of General Anaesthesia and Regional Anaesthesia in Terms of Mortality and Complications in Elderly Patients with Hip Fracture: A Nationwide Population-Based Study. *BMJ Open* **2019**, *9*, e029245. [CrossRef] [PubMed]
44. Rosa, R.G.; Falavigna, M.; Da Silva, D.B.; Sganzerla, D.; Santos, M.M.S.; Kochhann, R.; De Moura, R.M.; Eugênio, C.S.; Haack, T.D.S.R.; Barbosa, M.G.; et al. Effect of Flexible Family Visitation on Delirium Among Patients in the Intensive Care Unit: The ICU Visits Randomized Clinical Trial. *JAMA* **2019**, *322*, 216. [CrossRef] [PubMed]
45. Chu, C.-C.; Weng, S.-F.; Chen, K.-T.; Chien, C.-C.; Shieh, J.-P.; Chen, J.-Y.; Wang, J.-J. Propensity Score–Matched Comparison of Postoperative Adverse Outcomes between Geriatric Patients Given a General or a Neuraxial Anesthetic for Hip Surgery. *Anesthesiology* **2015**, *123*, 136–147. [CrossRef] [PubMed]
46. Neuman, M.D.; Rosenbaum, P.R.; Ludwig, J.M.; Zubizarreta, J.R.; Silber, J.H. Anesthesia Technique, Mortality, and Length of Stay After Hip Fracture Surgery. *JAMA* **2014**, *311*, 2508. [CrossRef] [PubMed]
47. Mounet, B.; Choquet, O.; Swisser, F.; Biboulet, P.; Bernard, N.; Bringuier, S.; Capdevila, X. Impact of Multiple Nerves Blocks Anaesthesia on Intraoperative Hypotension and Mortality in Hip Fracture Surgery Intermediate-Risk Elderly Patients: A Propensity Score-Matched Comparison with Spinal and General Anaesthesia. *Anaesth. Crit. Care Pain Med.* **2021**, *40*, 100924. [CrossRef]
48. Viderman, D.; Aubakirova, M.; Nabidollayeva, F.; Yegembayeva, N.; Bilotta, F.; Badenes, R.; Abdildin, Y. Effect of Ketamine on Postoperative Neurocognitive Disorders: A Systematic Review and Meta-Analysis. *J. Clin. Med.* **2023**, *12*, 4314. [CrossRef]
49. Sanfilippo, F.; La Via, L.; Tigano, S.; Morgana, A.; Rosa, V.; Astuto, M. Trial Sequential Analysis: The Evaluation of the Robustness of Meta-Analyses Findings and the Need for Further Research. *EuroMediterr. Biomed. J.* **2021**, *16*, 104–107. [CrossRef]
50. Cassai, A.D.; Pasin, L.; Boscolo, A.; Salvagno, M.; Navalesi, P. Trial Sequential Analysis: Plain and Simple. *Korean J. Anesthesiol.* **2020**, *74*, 363–365. [CrossRef]

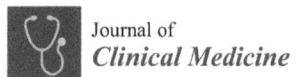

Journal of
Clinical Medicine

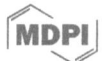

Systematic Review

The Impact of Transcutaneous Electrical Nerve Stimulation (TENS) on Acute Pain and Other Postoperative Outcomes: A Systematic Review with Meta-Analysis

Dmitriy Viderman [1,2,*], Fatima Nabidollayeva [3], Mina Aubakirova, Nurzhamal Sadir [1], Karina Tapinova [1], Ramil Tankacheyev [4] and Yerkin G. Abdildin [3]

[1] Department of Surgery, School of Medicine, Nazarbayev University, Astana 010000, Kazakhstan; mina.aubakirova@nu.edu.kz (M.A.); nurzhamal.sadir@nu.edu.kz (N.S.); karina.tapinova@nu.edu.kz (K.T.)
[2] Department of Anesthesiology, Intensive Care and Pain Medicine, National Research Oncology Center, Astana 010000, Kazakhstan
[3] Department of Mechanical and Aerospace Engineering, School of Engineering and Digital Sciences, Nazarbayev University, Astana 010000, Kazakhstan; fatima.nabidollayeva@nu.edu.kz (F.N.); yerkin.abdildin@nu.edu.kz (Y.G.A.)
[4] Department of Minimally Invasive Surgery, National Research Neurosurgery Center, Astana 010000, Kazakhstan; ramiltankacheyev@gmail.com
* Correspondence: drviderman@gmail.com

Citation: Viderman, D.; Nabidollayeva, F.; Aubakirova, M.; Sadir, N.; Tapinova, K.; Tankacheyev, R.; Abdildin, Y.G. The Impact of Transcutaneous Electrical Nerve Stimulation (TENS) on Acute Pain and Other Postoperative Outcomes: A Systematic Review with Meta-Analysis. *J. Clin. Med.* **2024**, *13*, 427. https://doi.org/10.3390/jcm13020427

Academic Editors: Felice Eugenio Agro, Giuseppe Pascarella, Fabio Costa and Kassiani Theodoraki

Received: 12 December 2023
Revised: 30 December 2023
Accepted: 5 January 2024
Published: 12 January 2024

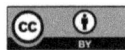
Abstract: This study aimed to investigate the efficacy and safety of transcutaneous electrical nerve stimulation (TENS) in postoperative acute pain control. PubMed, Scopus, and Cochrane Library were searched on 1–8 December 2022, for randomized controlled trials on the analgesic effects of TENS. The outcomes were pain intensity and opioid use (primary), and postoperative (PO) adverse events, blood pressure, and the duration of hospital stay (secondary); PROSPERO CRD42022333335. A total of 40 articles were included in the meta-analysis. Pain intensity at rest and during coughing for all types of surgeries combined was lower in the TENS group (standardized mean difference (SMD) = −0.51 [−0.61, −0.41], $p < 0.00001$, 29 studies, and −1.28 [−2.46, −0.09], p-value = 0.03, six studies, respectively). There was a statistically significant decrease in morphine requirements, as well as in the incidence of postoperative nausea and vomiting, dizziness, and pruritus. There was no difference between the groups in postoperative pain intensity during walking, in blood pressure, and only a borderline difference in the length of hospital stay. The subgroup analysis by surgery type did not show significant differences between the groups in pain severity at rest. Thus, TENS has a potential for pain control and postoperative recovery outcomes.

Keywords: acute pain; postoperative pain; transcutaneous electrical nerve stimulation; adverse events; hospital stay

1. Introduction

Acute pain is the most common symptom and patient complaint during the acute postoperative period. It can contribute to numerous unwanted physiological and pathological effects, such as cardiovascular activation, resulting in tachycardia, elevated blood pressure, and increased myocardial oxygen demand; it can also impair respiratory, endocrine, and other system impairments. For patients undergoing simple surgical procedures, pain is one of the most frequent reasons for overnight hospital stays [1,2]. Postoperative pain is also a major cause of prolonged hospitalization, leading to a potential increase in morbidity after surgery [1]. Improved pain management may enhance postoperative recovery and reduce morbidity [3].

Prescribing opioids for the management of moderate to severe pain often results in side effects, with the most common being nausea, vomiting, intestinal hypomotility, and respiratory depression. Interventional modalities of acute pain management, such as epidural analgesia, some newer plane blocks, including transversus abdominis plane block, erector spinae plane block, and quadratus lumborum block, can provide effective pain management but require experienced specialists and can result in complications, such as local anesthetic systemic toxicity [4–11]. Multimodal analgesia is usually recommended for pain reduction [3,12]. This approach may include opioids, regional analgesia, low-dose ketamine, and neurocognitive modalities [12]. Nonpharmacologic methods, including transcutaneous acupoint electrical stimulation (TENS) and "transcutaneous acupoint electrical stimulation" (TAES), have been studied to improve postoperative pain control and reduce analgesic drug requirements [13–15].

TENS is a physical method of controlled low-voltage electrical nerve stimulation used for the reduction of pain. The electricity is conducted by electrodes placed on the skin [16]. TENS is a non-invasive, portable, compact, easy-to-use, and safe method of pain control [16]. In the postoperative period, TENS is used as an add-on pain management modality to standard analgesics rather than a stand-alone modality. The sterile electrodes are applied parallel to the surgical incision, and additional electrodes are placed over the thoracic spinal nerves in the corresponding area [17]. The possible advantages of TENS in postoperative pain management include faster mobilization and improvement in deep respiratory function and coughing, which might also shorten the time to discharge from the hospital [17].

The original theory suggested that the activation of descending inhibitory pathways might be the mechanism of action of TENS. Previous studies also supported the mechanism of segmentally mediated inhibition. Therefore, TENS appears to activate both descending and segmental inhibition [18]. The analgesic effect of TENS is also produced by the pain gate control theory, which is characterized by an attenuation of the nociceptive stimulation of afferent fibers of large diameter in the dorsal horn [19]. Conventional TENS activates the A-α and A-β fibers, alleviating the pain. TENS also activates the endogenous opioid system. This activation is produced by high and low-frequency stimulations [20].

Two decades ago, a meta-analysis comprising 21 studies examined the use of TENS in various surgeries and its effect on opioid consumption [21]. However, more studies have been published over the past twenty years; therefore, there is a need for additional analysis of the currently available data. Recently, meta-analyses have been conducted on the analgesic effects of TENS in orthopedic [22], pulmonary [23], inguinal hernia repair [24], gynecological [25], and cardiothoracic surgical interventions [26]. A recent large meta-analysis of 381 studies, comprising almost 25,000 patients, studied the analgesic effect of TENS in all-cause pain [27]. The authors state that aggregating pain intensity data regardless of the underlying medical condition is appropriate, as there is a lack of conclusive evidence establishing a connection between TENS outcomes and factors such as pathology, pain characteristics, medical diagnoses, or clinical context [27]. While this study comprises all types of pain, including chronic and non-surgical, it is important to also examine the effect of TENS on acute postoperative pain.

While these previous publications have examined the effect of TENS on postoperative pain, the evidence regarding the impact of TENS on pain and other postoperative outcomes is still inconclusive. Therefore, the goal of this work was to assess the efficacy and safety of TENS in acute postoperative pain management, as well as its influence on opioid consumption, ICU and hospital stay, and the rate of postoperative complication. We hypothesize that the use of TENS in various surgeries lowers pain scores and opioid consumption and might be associated with a reduction in postoperative adverse events and hospital length of stay.

2. Materials and Methods

2.1. Protocol

We used the PRISMA guidelines [28] and the Cochrane Handbook for Systematic Reviews of Interventions [29]. The protocol was registered in the PROSPERO database (CRD42022333335). We searched for suitable articles in PubMed, Scopus, and the Cochrane

Library, published before December 2022. No gray literature was searched. We used the following search terms and combinations: ("transcutaneous electric nerve stimulation" OR ("transcutaneous" AND "electric" AND "nerve" AND "stimulation") OR "transcutaneous electric nerve stimulation" OR ("transcutaneous" AND "electrical" AND "nerve" AND "stimulation") OR "transcutaneous electrical nerve stimulation") OR "transcutaneous acupoint electrical stimulation" AND ("pain, postoperative" OR ("pain" AND "postoperative") OR "postoperative pain" OR ("postoperative" AND "pain")). The filters used were "randomized controlled trials" and "English language". No restrictions were used for the year or country of publication. Two authors independently worked on record screening and article searching. The search results retrieved from the mentioned databases were pooled in a spreadsheet, and duplicates were removed. Then, the two authors conducted the screening based on titles in accordance with the pre-specified inclusion criteria. The remaining articles were further screened based on the abstracts. Finally, the full texts were screened to identify those reporting the outcomes of interest. The final lists of articles were compared between the two authors. In case of disagreements, a third author was consulted to resolve the dispute.

2.2. Participants and Population
2.2.1. Inclusion Criteria

Patients: postoperative patients with no limitations on age, gender, or type of surgery.
Intervention: use of TENS.
Comparison: sham or no TENS (with standard postoperative pain management).
Outcomes: pain and other clinically important postoperative outcomes (please see below).
Study: randomized controlled trials (RCTs).

2.2.2. Exclusion Criteria

Types of studies: Study designs other than RCTs.
Outcomes: Studies not reporting the outcomes of interest.

2.3. Outcomes

The primary outcomes of our meta-analysis are postoperative (PO) pain (at rest, while walking, while coughing during a 72-h period postoperatively). The secondary outcomes were opioid consumption, postoperative adverse events, physiological parameters (blood pressure levels), and hospital stay duration (days).

2.4. Data Extraction and Statistical Methods

One author extracted and entered essential descriptive information (e.g., study goals and sample size). Another author extracted numeric data for meta-analysis from the studies. A third author further checked the descriptive and quantitative data, and disagreements were resolved by discussion. Data analysis was conducted using the software "Review Manager (RevMan) [Computer program]. Version 5.4. The Cochrane Collaboration, 2020". The random-effects model was employed for the meta-analysis, in anticipation of heterogeneity resulting from the combination of various types of surgeries, patient populations, and the different scales used to report the outcomes of interest. All outcome variables were continuous. In some instances, we estimated statistics from the reported data using established statistical methods [30,31]. The effect size was reported as the standardized mean difference (SMD), mean difference (MD), or risk ratio (RR), with a 95% confidence interval. The utilization of SMD allowed for the standardized comparison of effect sizes across diverse outcome measures, such as pain scores and opioid use, accommodating the varied scales and units of measurement employed in the included studies. The risk ratio was used for analyzing dichotomous outcomes, such as adverse events, providing a measure of the relative risk between the TENS and control groups. Statistical significance was reported at $p < 0.05$. Heterogeneity was measured using the I^2 statistic, which quantifies the proportion of total variation across studies due to heterogeneity. Additionally, the

p-value of Cochran's Q statistic was considered to evaluate the statistical significance of observed heterogeneity. A significance level of 0.1 was employed to determine whether the observed heterogeneity was statistically significant. Sensitivity analyses were performed for each outcome by running the model with the elimination of studies one by one and were reported only if the results were sensitive.

2.5. Assessment of the Methodological Quality and the Publication Bias

Two authors independently assessed the methodological quality. The Cochrane Risk of Bias tool 2.0 [32] was utilized to evaluate the methodological quality of the studies. The risk of bias was categorized as "high", "low", or "medium/some concerns", based on the provided description of randomization and blinding procedures, as well as the reporting of results. Furthermore, we assessed the certainty of evidence using the Grading of Recommendations Assessment, Development, and Evaluation (GRADE) [33]. Five outcomes (pain at rest at 24 h, morphine consumption at 24 h, PONV, pruritus, and hospital length of stay) were evaluated for upgrading or downgrading based on the risk of bias, imprecision, inconsistency, and indirectness. Each of these outcomes received a certainty of evidence grading ranging from "very low" to "high". Additionally, we conducted a comprehensive assessment of publication bias utilizing both funnel plots and Egger's regression test.

3. Results

3.1. Article Search Results

In total, 182 articles were initially identified (Figure 1). Of them, 89 duplicates were removed. Subsequently, 93 RCTs were screened. After screening the titles and abstracts, 53 articles were excluded. Finally, a total of 40 articles [2,13,34–71] with 2265 (TENS—1137, control—1128) patients were included in the meta-analysis (Table 1).

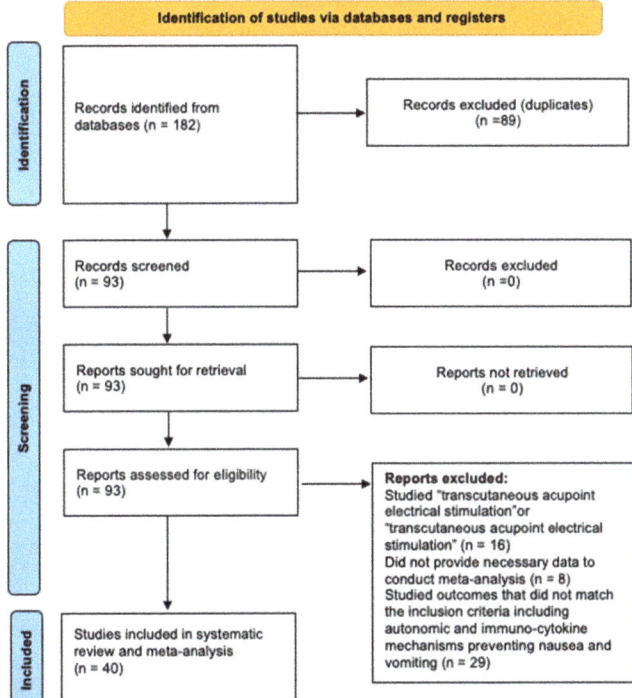

Figure 1. PRISMA diagram.

Table 1. Study characteristics. Abbreviations: RoM, range of motion; TKA, total knee arthroplasty; VAS, visual analog scale; LAS, linear analog scale; N, number; PONV, postoperative vomiting and nausea; TENS, transcutaneous electrical nerve stimulation; QoR, quality of recovery; NRS, numeric rating scale; TEAS, transcutaneous acupoint stimulation; QoL, quality of life [2,13,34–71].

Author, Year, Country	Study Goals	Age	N of Patients: Total (TENS/Control); % Male	% Male (TENS/Control)	Groups	Diagnosis	Comorbidities	Type of Surgery	The Timing of TENS	Method of Pain Measurement	Study Conclusions
Beckwee, 2017, Belgium [41]	Pain, knee RoM, analgesic use	71.8 (7.3) 72.9 (7.6)	53 (25/28)	32%/39.3%	TENS Sham	-	-	TKA	40 min	100 mm VAS before and after, daily	No effects on pain
Forogh, 2017, Iran [56]	Pain, IKDC, RoM	26 (4.1) 26.31 (4.33)	70 (35/35)	100%	TENS No TENS, both groups exercise	Injury to the ACL	-	Post-anterior cruciate ligament reconstruction	20 sessions, 4 weeks, 35 min/day	100 mm VAS	No effect on knee function and pain
Asgari, 2018, Iran [37]	Pain, fentanyl use, PONV	31.35 (4.89) 31.15 (6.28)	80 (40/40)	0%	TENS No TENS, 50 mg fentanyl	Ectopic pregnancy, infertility, ovarian cysts, ovarian torsion	-	Laparoscopic Gynecologic Surgery	20 min for patients who complained of pain	10-cm VAS before, and 5, 10, 20, 30 min after treatment	TENS is not superior to fentanyl for pain relief
Bjersa, 2014, Sweden [62]	Pain, QoR-40, extra analgesia use, EDA infusion rate, total TENS use time	69.1 65.5	20 (9/11)	56%/73%	TENS Sham	-	-	Pancreatic resection: Ad Modum Whipple pancreaticoduodenectomy	30 min sessions; for 24 h post-op	Pain-O-Meter, estimation on 100-mm scale	Supports use of high-frequency TENS
Bjersa, 2015, Sweden [38]	Pain, QoR-40, total analgesia use, time of TENS use	67.9 (11.6) 74.1 (10.3)	28 (15/13)	53%/86%	TENS Sham	Colon diseases and malignancies, unknown	-	Open colon resection	No time limits; each session—30 min; for 24 h post-op	Pain-O-Meter, estimation on 100-mm scale	Benefits of TENS
Cuschieri, 1985, UK [63]	Pain, morphine use, ABG	51 57	106 (53/53)	43%/40%	TENS Sham	-	-	Abdominal surgery	3 days post-op	LAS, before + after twice daily for 3 days	Results do not support TENS use
Galli, 2014, Brazil [57]	Pain	44.32 (9.98) 44.22 (8.21)	74 (37/37)	57%/38%	TENS Sham	Healthy kidney donors	HTN, asthma, gastritis, hypothyroidism	Open nephrectomy	For 1 h during first post-op day	NRS before and after	TENS decreases pain and increases max expiratory pressure

18

Table 1. Cont.

Author, Year, Country	Study Goals	Age	N of Patients: Total (TENS/Control); % Male	% Male (TENS/Control)	Groups	Diagnosis	Comorbidities	Type of Surgery	The Timing of TENS	Method of Pain Measurement	Study Conclusions
Hamza, 1999, USA [67]	PCA demands and doses, sedation, fatigue, discomfort, pain, nausea, side effects	43 (11) 44 (11) 45 (10) 43 (9)	100 (25/25/25/25)	0%	PCA + sham PCA + low-frequency TENS PCA + high-frequency TENS PCA + mixed-frequency TENS	-	-	Major gynecological procedures	Every 2 h during the day	100 mm VAS at baseline, 24, 48 h	TENS decreases post-op opioid analgesic use and opioid-related side effects
Laitinen, 1991, Finland [68]	Pain, BP, HR, RR, side effects	63.4 (7.8) 50.2 (8.6) 56.6 (11.5) 61.4 (8.4) 52.2 (8.4) 40.6 (11.4) 49.6 (16.9) 46.9 (14)	60 (10/10/20/20)	20%/0%/0%/0%/3%	Control Indomethacin Low-frequency TENS + indomethacin High-frequency TENS + indomethacin	Cholecystitis	-	Cholecystectomy	16 h	No/mild/moderate/n at rest, MMSE, PONV, medsevere every 4 h	Neither indomethacin nor TENS reduce the post-operative opiate requirement.
Rakel, 2003, USA [60]	Pain, walking function, vital capacity	20–77 40 (15)	33	48%	Pharmacologic analgesia + TENS Pharmacologic + sham TENS Pharmacologic only	-	End-stage renal disease, diabetes	-	15 min, 2–4 h between the sessions	NRS 0–20	Reduces pain and increases walking function post-op
Silva, 2012, Brazil [13]	Pain, PONV	52 (14) 44 (16)	42 (21/21)	7%	TENS Sham TENS	Cholecystitis	-	Laparoscopic cholecystectomy	30 min during 24h post-op	11-point VNS, VAS (0–10)	Decreases pain and PONV
Yu, 2020, China [52]	QoR, pain at rest, MMSE, PONV, medication use	48.5 (16.2) 45.9 (17.5)	60 (30/30)	0%	TEAS Sham TEAS	-	-	Gynecological laparoscopic surgery	30 min before anesthesia	100 mm VAS	Improves QoR, MMSE; reduces pain, PONV
Zhang, 2017, China [53]	Pain, bladder spasm episodes	64.5 (54–79)	66 (30/36)	100%	TENS No TENS	BPH, bladder disease	-	Bladder or prostate surgery	3 days post-op, each session for 60 min	VAS 0–10	Relieves post-op bladder spasms
Zhang, 2018, China [54]	Pain, time to first: defecation, flatulence, diet; LOS, HRV	68 (1.4) 64 (2.6)	42 (21/21)	86%/71%	TEAS Sham TEAS	GI cancers	-	Open abdominal surgery for cancers	1 h, twice daily, 3 d	VAS 0–10	Improves major post-op symptoms

Table 1. *Cont.*

Author, Year, Country	Study Goals	Age	N of Patients: Total (TENS/Control); % Male	% Male (TENS/Control)	Groups	Diagnosis	Comorbidities	Type of Surgery	The Timing of TENS	Method of Pain Measurement	Study Conclusions
Chiu, 1999, Taiwan [42]	Pain, total PCA morphine use, N of nurse calls for analgesia	53.1 (2.7), 56.0 (3.1)	60: (30/30)	75%	TENS on acupoints, TENS on sham acupoints	Symptomatic hemorrhoids	-	Hemorrhoidectomy	Postoperative, 2 times a day	0–10	Complications—hemoperi-cardium, better pain relief
Elboim-Gabyzon, 2019, Israel [43]	Pain, FAC, physical performance	78.06 (8.45), 80.26 (9.83)	41: (18/23)	13%/33%	TENS Sham TENS	Intertrochanteric or sub-trochanteric fracture	Yes	Hip fracture surgery	Postoperative	NRS 0–10	Pain relief
Benedetti, 1997, Italy [66]	Time to analgesia, total medication use, pain	-	103 106 112	Not given	TENS Sham TENS No TENS	Empyema, myasthenia gravis	-	Posterolateral thoracotomy, muscle-sparing thoracotomy, costotomy, sternotomy, and video-assisted thoracoscopy	1 h post-op, 1 h rest interval, 1h more	NRS 0–10	Useful for mild to moderate pain; ineffective for severe pain
Engen, 2015, USA [44]	Pain, analgesia use, patient satisfaction	61.5 (11.21), 61.8 (13.13)	56: (28/28)	30%/55%	TENS + opioids Opioids only	-	-	Thoracoscopic surgery	48 h post-operatively	VAS 0–10	No effect on pain or morphine use
Erden, 2016, Turkey [36]	Pain, analgesic use	54.9 (13.3), 50.0 (12.7)	40: (20/20)	70%/80%	TENS No TENS	Lung cancer	Chronic disease	Posterolateral thoracotomy	Postoperative 30 min	VAS	Reduces pain
Erdogan, 2005, Turkey [46]	Pain, FEV1, FVC, PaO2, PaCO2, doses of analgesia, sedation, side effects	55.6 (11.9), 52.93 (11.48)	116 (60/56)	63%/57%	TENS No TENS	Lung cancer	-	Posterolateral thoracotomy	For 20 min at 3-h intervals for 3 days	VAS 0–10	Routine use recommended
Ferreira, 2011, Brazil [40]	Pain	49 (14), 55.0 (14.9)	30: (15/15)	67%/53%	TENS Sham TENS	Lung cancer	-	Thoracotomy	Second post-op day	VAS 10 cm	Reduces pain severity
Fiorelli, 2011, Italy [2]	Cytokines, pain, respiratory function, medication usage	64 (1), 64 (4.1)	50: (25/25)	74%/61%	TENS Sham TENS	Lung cancer	-	Standard posterolateral thoracotomy	48 h post-op, 30 min	VAS 0–10	Reduces pain

Table 1. *Cont.*

Author, Year, Country	Study Goals	Age	N of Patients: Total (TENS/Control); % Male	% Male (TENS/Control)	Groups	Diagnosis	Comorbidities	Type of Surgery	The Timing of TENS	Method of Pain Measurement	Study Conclusions
Gregorini, 2010, Brazil [58]	Pain, respiratory function	59.9 (10.3)	25: (13/12)	72%	TENS / Sham TENS	-	-	Elective cardiac surgery	Third post-op day	VAS	Reduces pain
Jahangirifard, 2018, Iran [61]	Pain, respiratory function, narcotics use, drain secretions, ICU LoS, N requests for chest radiographs	58.4 (8.1), 60.1 (6.6)	100: (50/50)	50%/50%	TENS / Sham TENS	-	-	Elective coronary artery bypass	Post-op 30 min every 4 h	VAS 0–10	Reduces pain, better pulmonary function
Lima, 2011, Brazil [39]	Pain, MIP, MEP	54.2 / 55.1	20 (10/10)	50%	TENS / No TENS	CAD	-	CABG	30 min, 3 times a day, 3 h each	VAS 0–10	Reduces pain; increase in respiratory muscle strength
Navarathnam, 1984, Australia [65]	Pulmonary function, analgesic use, atelectasis, pain	56.4 (39–67) / 52.2 (17–69)	31 (14/17)	86%/77%	TENS / Sham TENS	CAD, valve disease	-	CABG, AV replacement, MV replacement	-	Digital scoring system (1–5)	May be of benefit in post-op pain relief
Sezen, 2017, Turkey [50]	Post-op pain, complications	55.13 (14.63), 58.86 (11.82)	87: (43/44)	74%/68%	TENS / Sham TENS	-	-	Thoracotomy	8 h post-op	VAS 0–10	No effect on hospital stay, complications; safe pain management
Solak, 2007, Turkey [69]	Pain, pulmonary function	47.3 (11.7) / 53.72 (12.6)	40 (20/20)	70%/90%	TENS / PCA	-	-	Posterolateral thoracotomy	4 h post-op	VAS, Prince Henry score	Better pain relief than PCA
Stubbing, 1988, UK [70]	Analgesic use, time to oral analgesia, antiemetic use, LoS, pulmonary function	54 (17.8) / 53 (15.7)	40 (20/20)	65%/75%	TENS + IM papaveretum / IM papaveretum alone	-	-	Thoracotomy	For 48 h post-op	0–4	Lower PONV, no effect on analgesia use, peak expiratory flow rate

Table 1. *Cont.*

Author, Year, Country	Study Goals	Age	N of Patients: Total (TENS/Control); % Male	% Male (TENS/Control)	Groups	Diagnosis	Comorbidities	Type of Surgery	The Timing of TENS	Method of Pain Measurement	Study Conclusions
Kara, 2011, Turkey [48]	Pain, function, depression, side effects	45.62 (10.59) 47.60 (13.75)	54 (25/29)	40%/55%	TENS + PCA PCA only	-	-	Open lumbar discectomy	Twice for 30–40 min, 3–4 h interval	Horizontal 100 mm VAS	Reduces side effects, analgesic use, activity-related pain
McCallum, 1988, UK [64]	Morphine use	44.6 (9.1), 45.7 (11.7)	20: (10/10)	50%/20%	TENS Sham TENS	-	-	Lumbar laminectomy	12 h prior to surgery	-	No effect on pain
Parseliunas, 2020, Lithuania [49]	Pain, analgesics use	61.77 (10.84), 61.08 (12.51)	80: (40/40)	100%	TENS Sham TENS	Unilateral inguinal hernia	-	Open inguinal hernia repair	Post-op	100 mm VAS	Reduces post-op pain
Smedley, 1988, UK [51]	Pain, analgesic use, peak expiratory flow	57 (21–83) 55 (24–78)	62 (34/28)	100%	TENS Sham TENS	Inguinal hernia	-	Inguinal hernia repair	48 h post-op	LAS	No differences
Chen, 2021, China [55]	Pain, pain attacks, N/amount analgesic drugs, changes in gene expression	73%: 20–35	70 (35/35)	0%	TENS + analgesic drugs Analgesic drugs only	-	-	Elective C-section	24 h post-op, 30 min each	10 cm VAS	Reduces pain, N pain attacks, analgesic use, and expression of PNMT gene
Kurata, 2022, USA [47]	Opioid use, pain, patient satisfaction, LOS, adverse events	31 (6) 32 (6) 31 (6)	180 (60/60/60) ITT	0%	TENS Sham TENS No TENS	Obstetric	Prior c-section, other uterine incision	C-section	30 min post-op, until discharge, PCA	0–10 Likert scale	No effect on opioid use, pain, LOS
da Silva, 2015, Brazil [35]	Pain, analgesic use, adverse effects, quality of pain, treatment success, patient satisfaction	25 27	42 (21/21)	100%	TENS Sham TENS	-	-	Liposuction	30 min post-op	-	Effective in adjunction to analgesics for pain
Erden, 2022, Turkey [45]	Pain, patient satisfaction	57.1 (10.88) 56.9 (10.2)	80 (40/40)	0%	TENS No TENS	Breast cancer	Chronic diseases	Mastectomy	2 times for 20 min	NRS 0–10	Useful analgesic method

Table 1. *Cont.*

Author, Year, Country	Study Goals	Age	N of Patients: Total (TENS/Control); % Male	% Male (TENS/Control)	Groups	Diagnosis	Comorbidities	Type of Surgery	The Timing of TENS	Method of Pain Measurement	Study Conclusions
Ilfeld, 2021, USA [34]	Opioid use, pain, QoL	56.8 (15.8) 55.4 (15.9)	65 (31/34)	52%/50%	TENS Sham TENS	ACL injury, rotator cuff injury, hallux valgus, ankle arthrodesis, arthroplasty	-	Major foot/ankle surgery, anterior cruciate ligament reconstruction, rotator cuff repair	Up to 14 d post-op, daily	Average daily NRS 0–10	Reduces pain and opioid use, no systemic side effects
Mahure, 2017, USA [59]	Anesthetic use, pain	60.5 (11.1) 56.4 (12.2)	37 (21/16)	53%/44%	TENS Sham TENS	-	-	Arthroscopic rotator cuff repair	-	VAS	Less pain, opioid use
Wang, 2014, China [71]	Intraoperative remifentanil use, side effects	43.1 (15.0) 39.9 (15.7	60 (30/30)	53%/63%	TEAS Sham TEAS	-	-	Sinusotomy	30 min before anesthesia	-	Less incidence of side-effects

3.2. Assessment of Methodological Quality

Regarding methodological quality, 10 studies had a low risk of bias, while 29 studies were assessed as having "some concerns" regarding the risk of bias. One study had a high risk of bias. The detailed results of the quality analysis are presented in Table 2 [2,13,34–71].

Table 2. Risk of Bias table. "+" low risk of bias; "?" some concerns; "-" high risk of bias.

First Author, Year	1	2	3	4	5	6
Asgari 2018 [37]	+	?	+	+	+	?
Beckwee 2017 [41]	?	+	+	+	+	?
Benedetti 1997 [66]	?	?	+	+	+	?
Bjersa 2014 [62]	+	?	+	+	+	?
Bjersa 2015 [38]	+	?	+	+	+	?
Chen 2021 [55]	?	?	+	+	+	?
Chiu 1999 [42]	+	?	+	+	+	?
Cuschieri 1985 [63]	?	+	+	+	+	?
da Silva 2015 [35]	+	?	?	+	+	?
Elboim-Gabyzon 2019 [43]	+	+	+	+	+	+
Engen 2015 [44]	?	?	+	+	+	?
Erden 2022 [45]	+	+	-	-	+	+
Erden 2016 [36]	+	?	+	+	+	?
Erdogan 2005 [46]	?	+	+	+	+	?
Ferreira 2011 [40]	?	?	+	+	+	?
Fiorelli 2011 [2]	+	+	+	+	+	+
Forogh 2017 [56]	+	+	+	+	+	+
Galli 2015 [57]	+	+	+	+	+	+
Gregorini 2010 [58]	+	?	+	+	+	?
Hamza 1999 [67]	+	?	?	+	+	?
Ilfeld 2021 [34]	+	+	+	+	+	+
Jahangirifard 2018 [61]	?	+	+	+	+	?
Kara 2011 [48]	+	?	+	+	+	?
Kurata 2022 [47]	+	+	+	+	+	+
Laitinen 1991 [68]	?	?	+	+	+	?
Lima 2011 [39]	-	?	?	?	?	-
Mahure 2017 [59]	+	?	+	?	+	?
McCallum 1988 [64]	?	+	+	+	+	?
Navarathnam 1984 [65]	?	?	+	+	+	?
Parseliunas 2020 [49]	+	+	+	+	+	+
Rakel 2003 [60]	?	?	+	+	+	?
Sezen 2017 [50]	?	?	+	+	+	?
Silva 2012 [13]	+	?	+	+	+	?
Smedley 1988 [51]	+	?	+	+	+	?

Table 2. *Cont.*

First Author, Year	1	2	3	4	5	6
Solak 2007 [69]	?	?	+	+	+	?
Stubbing 1988 [70]	?	?	+	+	+	?
Wang 2014	+	+	+	+	+	+
Yu 2020 [52]	+	+	+	+	+	+
Zhang 2017 [53]	+	?	+	+	+	?
Zhang 2018 [54]	?	?	+	+	+	?

1. Risk of bias arising from the randomization process. 2. Risk of bias arising from deviations from the intended interventions. 3. Risk of bias arising from missing outcome data. 4. Risk of bias arising from the measurement of the outcome. 5. Risk of bias arising from the selection of the reported results. 6. Overall risk of bias.

3.3. Pain at Rest

The forest plot in Figure 2 illustrates the pain intensity at rest measured immediately after surgery, 24 h post-surgery, and at various intervals. The overall model effect favors TENS over the control, indicating a standardized mean difference (SMD) on a 0-10 scale with a 95% CI of −0.79 [−1.21, −0.36], with a *p*-value less than 0.00001. However, it is important to note that the model shows substantial heterogeneity (I^2 = 94%). The TENS group comprises 891 patients, while the control group consists of 876 patients. One study [72] was excluded from the meta-analysis due to the absence of a reported sample standard deviation.

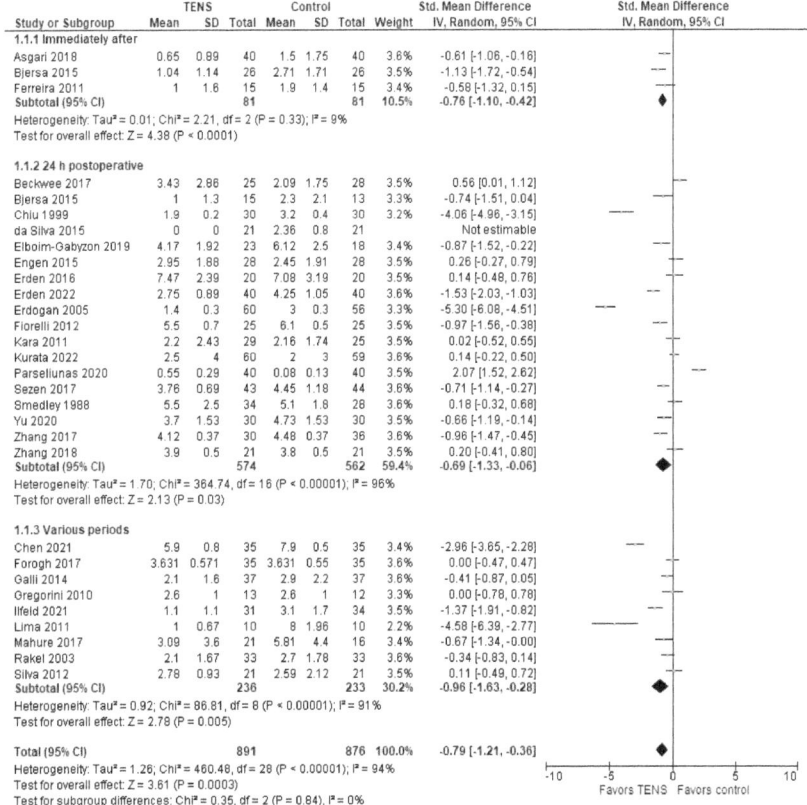

Figure 2. Pain at rest [2,13,34–42,44,45,47–60].

Subgroup analysis further reinforces the superiority of TENS over the control across all three subgroups ('immediately after surgery', '24 h after surgery', and 'various periods'), although with considerable heterogeneity for the latter two ($I^2 = 96\%$ and $I^2 = 91\%$, respectively). In the 'immediately after surgery' subgroup, the SMD with a 95% CI is -0.76 $[-1.10, -0.42]$, with a highly significant p-value < 0.0001, $I^2 = 9\%$. In the primary (24 h postoperative) subgroup, the SMD with a 95% CI is -0.69 $[-1.33, -0.06]$, with a p-value of 0.03, $I^2 = 96\%$. The third subgroup, covering varied measurement times, such as 'after TENS' [13], '12 h postoperative' [59], 'postoperative day 3' [58], 'postoperative day 7' [34], '4 weeks postoperative' [56], and instances with no provided information [39,55,57,60], shows a significant SMD with a 95% CI of -0.96 $[-1.63, -0.28]$, with a p-value of 0.005, $I^2 = 91\%$. These results indicate statistically significant improvements in pain intensity for the TENS group in all the measured periods.

3.4. Pain at Rest for Specific Types of Surgeries 24 h PO

The pain intensity at rest, measured 24 h after three different types of surgeries (abdominal, thoracic, and orthopedic), is presented in the forest plot below (Figure 3). The overall effect of the model shows no significant difference between TENS and control (SMD on a 0–10 scale with a 95% CI = -0.56 $[-1.23, 0.11]$, p-value = 0.10), and the model shows substantial heterogeneity with the value of $I^2 = 96\%$. However, the result is sensitive to the exclusion of the study by Parseliunas (2020), in which case the model favors the TENS group. The total number of patients in the TENS group is 518, and 519 in the control group. Two studies [35,45], representing the results for plastic and breast surgery, respectively, were excluded.

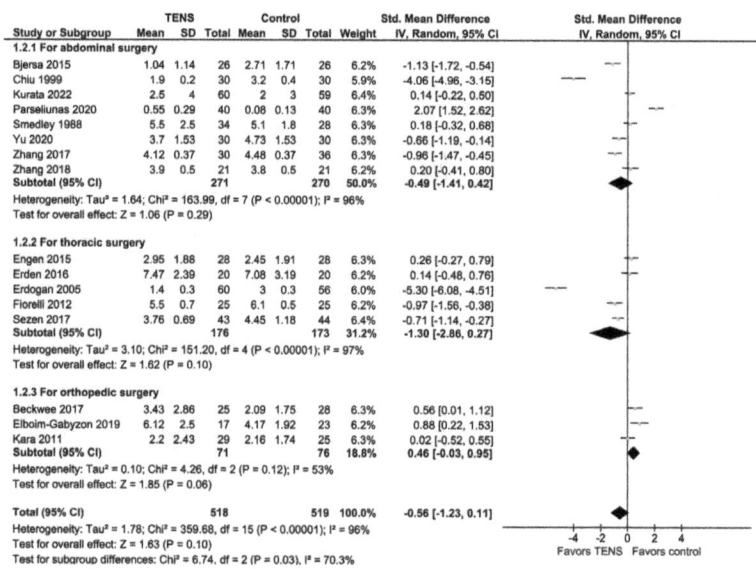

Figure 3. Pain at rest 24 h after different surgeries [2,36,38,41–44,46–54].

In terms of subgroup analysis, the model shows no significant difference between the TENS and control groups. The 'For abdominal surgery' subgroup yielded an SMD of -0.49 $[-1.41, 0.42]$, p-value = 0.29; the 'For thoracic surgery' subgroup yielded an SMD of -1.30 $[-2.86, 0.27]$, p-value = 0.10; and the "For orthopedic surgery" subgroup yielded an SMD of 0.46 $[-0.03, 0.95]$, p-value = 0.06.

3.5. Pain while Walking (POD 1, POD 2)

The forest plot in Figure 4 illustrates the pain intensity while walking measured 24 h and 48 h after surgery. The overall effect of the model does not favor TENS over the control (SMD with a 95% CI: 0.61 [−1.52, 2.74], *p*-value = 0.57). This result is sensitive to the exclusion of the study by Elboim-Gabyzon et al., 2019 [43]. The model shows considerable heterogeneity (I^2 = 96%), which is likely attributed to the limited number of included studies. Parseliunas et al., 2020 [49] reported pain while walking values for postoperative day 1 (POD 1), whereas Elboim-Gabyzon et al., 2019 [43] reported them for POD 2.

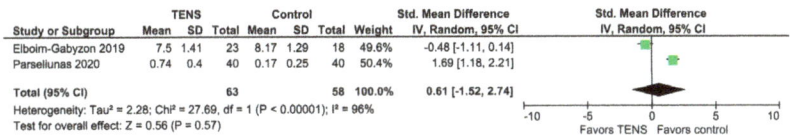

Figure 4. Pain while walking (POD 1, POD 2) [43,49].

3.6. Pain at Coughing (POD 1, POD 3)

The overall effect of the model favors the TENS group over the control group (SMD with a 95% CI: −1.28 [−2.46, −0.09], *p*-value = 0.03) (Figure 5). This result is statistically significant but sensitive to the exclusion of some studies [45,46,61]. Subgroup analysis reveals no significant difference between the groups. It is important to note that one study [57] did not provide the time of measurements, and as a result, we included it in the POD 3 subgroup.

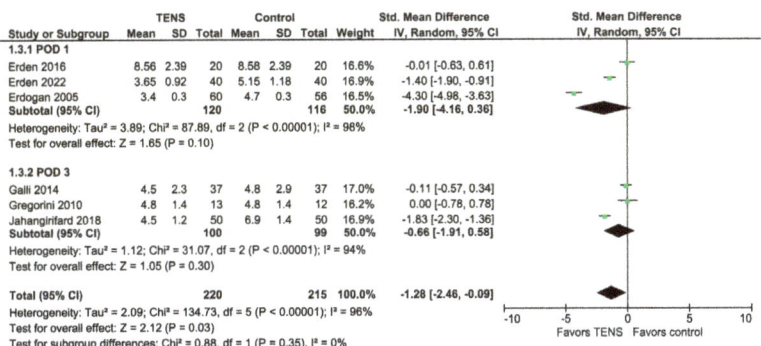

Figure 5. Pain at coughing (POD1, POD 3) [36,45,46,57,58,61].

3.7. Morphine Requirements (mg)

One study [66] reported ketorolac intake (mg), and we adjusted the values by multiplying them by 0.4, following the recommendation of the American Pain Society in 2003 and 2008 (https://cdn-links.lww.com/permalink/jpsn/a/jpsn_4_2_2015_04_23_manworren_jpsn-d-14-00050r2_sdc1.pdf (accessed on 15 December 2022)). Another study [38] reported IV oxycodone (mg) consumption, and we used a conversion factor of 1.5. Finally, one study [62] reported IV morphine consumption at 24 h; however, there was not enough information about the units (mL in the Table, but mg in the text), so we did not include this study in the analysis (the results were not sensitive to the values from this study).

Some studies [42,47,66] did not explicitly report the time of measurement, so we included them in the 'No time info' subgroup. The majority of the studies reported morphine requirements within 24 h after surgery ('POD 1' subgroup). One study [61] was excluded due to the absence of information about the sample standard deviation.

The overall effect of the model favors TENS over control (MD with a 95% CI: −7.82 [−13.48, −2.16], *p*-value < 0.00001) (Figure 6). However, this result is sensitive to the exclusion of a study by Chen 2021 [55]. Broken down, on POD1, the use of TENS decreased morphine use by 15.64 mg [−26.69, −4.58], p-value = 0.006, I^2 = 97%. In the "no time" subgroup, morphine use was decreased by 6.28 mg (−6.28 [−10.12, −2.43], p-value = 0.001, I^2 = 90%) in the TENS group.

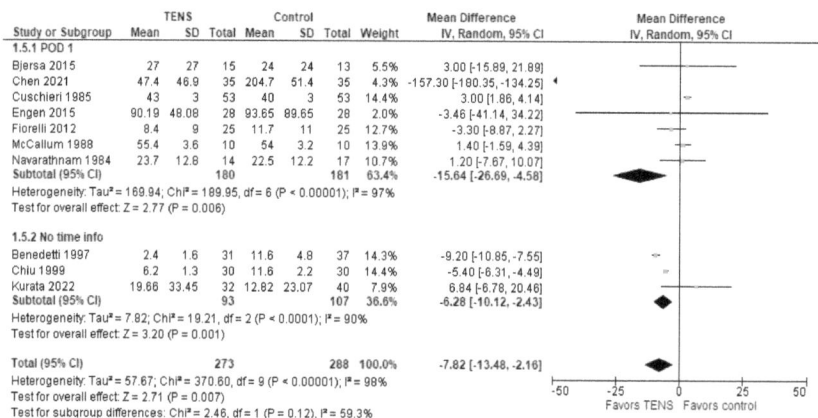

Figure 6. Postoperative morphine requirements (mg) [2,38,42,44,47,55,63–66].

3.8. Postoperative Nausea and Vomiting

The overall effect of the model favors the TENS group over the control group (the risk ratio (RR) with a 95% CI: 0.52 [0.30, 0.93], p-value = 0.03; I^2 = 51%) (Figure 7). It should be noted that the studies primarily reported the incidences of PONV on postoperative day 1 (POD 1) and postoperative day 2 (POD 2), but several studies did not explicitly report the time of measurement [13,35,46].

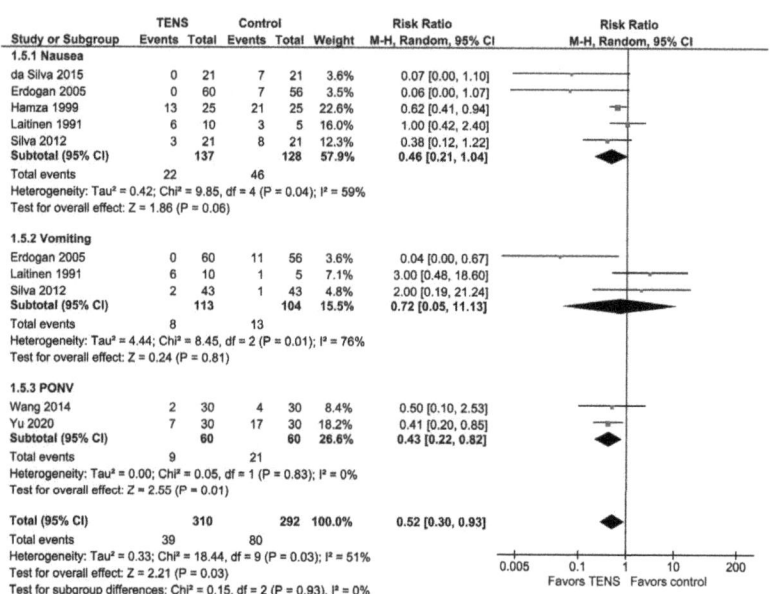

Figure 7. PO nausea and vomiting [13,35,46,52,67,68,71].

The subgroup analysis indicates that the model favors the TENS group over the control group in two subgroups, namely 'nausea' and 'PONV'.

3.9. Other Adverse Events (Dizziness and Pruritus)

The overall effect of the model favors TENS over control (RR with a 95% CI: 0.42 [0.29, 0.61], *p*-value < 0.00001, I^2 = 0%) (Figure 8). The model supports TENS over control in both subgroups: 'dizziness' and 'pruritus'. Specifically, for dizziness, the RR for the TENS group is 0.39 [0.23, 0.66], *p*-value = 0.0005, I^2 = 0%, 2 studies, 110 patients. For pruritus, the RR for the TENS group is 0.44 [0.26, 0.76], *p*-value = 0.003, I^2 = 0%, 3 studies, 226 patients.

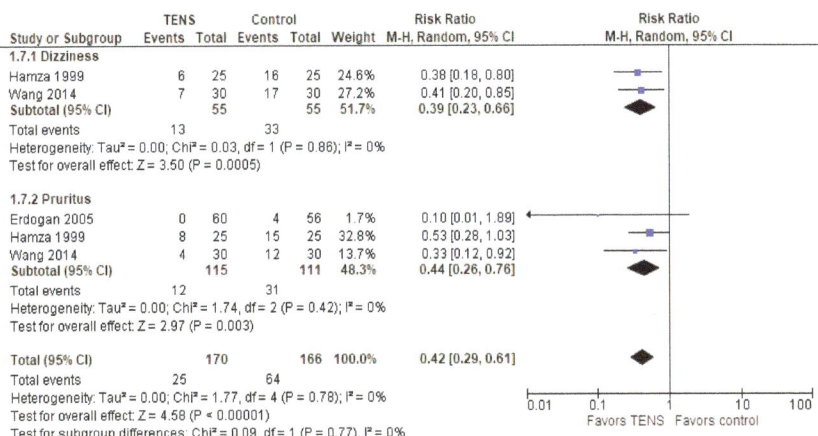

Figure 8. Other adverse events [46,67,71].

3.10. Hospital Stay Duration (Days)

The model shows no significant difference between TENS and control (MD with a 95% CI: −1.16 [−2.35, 0.02], *p*-value = 0.05; I^2 = 94%) (Figure 9). The result is sensitive to the exclusion of any of these three studies: Erdogan 2005, Solak 2007, or Stubbing 1998, in which case, the model favors TENS.

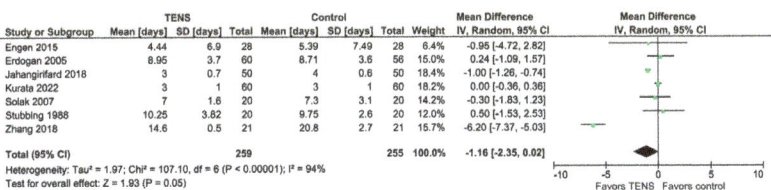

Figure 9. Hospital stay duration (days) [44,46,47,54,61,69,70].

3.11. Blood Pressure Postoperatively (mmHg)

The model indicates no significant difference between TENS and control (MD with a 95% CI: 0.98 [−1.20, 3.16], *p*-value = 0.38; I^2 = 0%) (Figure 10). Sezen et al., 2017 [50] reported the blood pressure values for postoperative day 1 (POD 1), and Gregorini et al., 2010 [58] reported these for postoperative day 3 (POD 3).

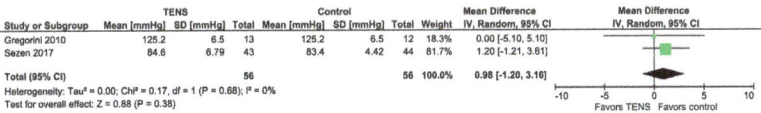

Figure 10. Blood pressure PO (mmHg) [50,58].

3.12. Publication Bias

Our findings from the analyses using the funnel plots and Egger's regression test did not indicate substantial evidence of publication bias in the studies included in our meta-analysis regarding pain intensity.

The funnel plot below for the pain intensity at rest (Figure 11) demonstrates a spread of study outcomes that resembles a slightly asymmetric distribution. This slight asymmetry could be attributed to the nature of the random effects model, accounting for potential heterogeneity among the included studies.

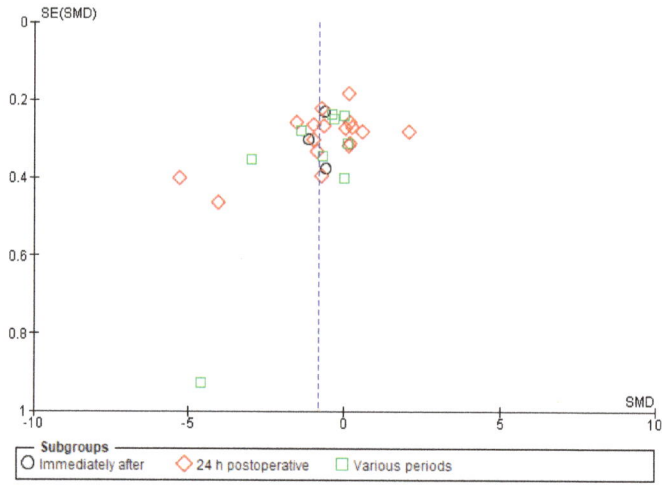

Figure 11. Funnel plot for pain at rest, the random effects model.

In contrast, the funnel plot under the fixed effect model (Figure 12) illustrates a more symmetric distribution of study outcomes. However, it is important to note that the fixed effect model assumes homogeneity across studies, which might not accurately represent the true variability seen in the data.

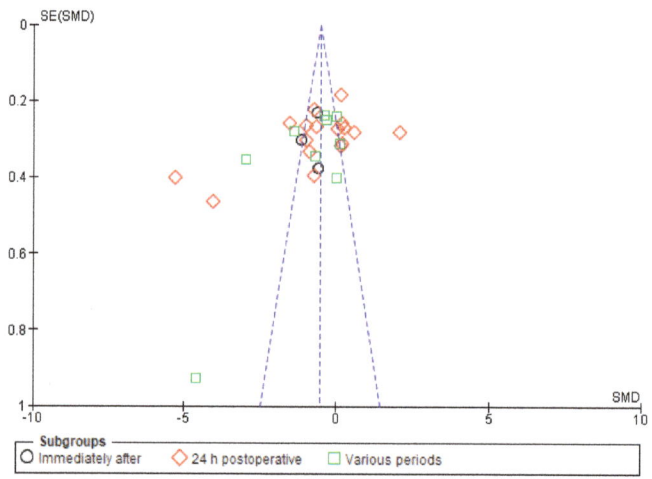

Figure 12. Funnel plot for pain at rest, the fixed effects model.

3.13. Certainty of Evidence

Table 3 provides the certainty of the evidence for five outcomes (pain at rest at 24 h, morphine consumption at 24 h, PONV, postoperative adverse events, and hospital length of stay). The certainty of evidence ranges from "very low" to "moderate". The evidence profile (Table 4) contains information regarding the quality of evidence evaluation and the summary of findings for each of the studied outcomes.

Table 3. Summary of findings. ⊕⊕⊕⊕ high quality of evidence, ⊕⊕⊕⊖ moderate quality of evidence, ⊕⊕⊖⊖ low quality of evidence, ⊕⊖⊖⊖ very low quality of evidence. Population: Patients undergoing various surgeries. Settings: In-hospital. Intervention: Use of TENS. Comparison: No TENS [2,13,34–71].

Outcomes	Risk Ratio (95% CI)	(Standardized) Mean Difference [95% CI]	N of Participants (Studies)	Certainty of the Evidence (GRADE)
Pain at rest, 24 h (0–10)	-	−0.69 [−1.33, −0.06]	1136 (18)	⊕⊖⊖⊖ Very low [a]
Morphine requirements, 24 h (mg)	-	−15.64 [−26.69, −4.58]	361 (7)	⊕⊖⊖⊖ Very low [b]
Postoperative nausea	0.46 [0.21, 1.04]	-	265 (5)	⊕⊕⊖⊖ Low [c]
Pruritus	0.44 [0.26, 0.76]	-	226 (3)	⊕⊕⊕⊖ Moderate [d]
Hospital stay duration (days)	-	−1.16 [−2.35, 0.02]	514 (7)	⊕⊕⊖⊖ Low [e]

[a] For three studies, the randomization method was unclear. Four studies were not blinded, and for two, blinding was unclear. There was considerable heterogeneity, wide variance of point estimates, and some confidence intervals did not overlap. [b] Four studies did not specify randomization procedures. One study was not blinded, and one study did not mention blinding. There was considerable heterogeneity, wide variance of point estimates, and some confidence intervals did not overlap. The confidence interval of the pooled effect crossed the no-difference line. [c] For two studies, the randomization method was unclear. Two studies were not blinded, and for two studies, blinding was unclear. There was moderate heterogeneity. The overall risk ratio was lower than 0.5; therefore, the outcome was upgraded. [d] For one study, the randomization method was unclear, for another, blinding was unclear. The overall risk ratio was lower than 0.5. [e] Four studies did not properly describe the randomization process. One study was not blinded, and two did not mention blinding. There was considerable heterogeneity and a wide variance of point estimates.

Table 4. The evidence profile (the quality of evidence evaluation and the summary of findings for each of the studied outcomes).

	Pain at Rest, 24 h	Morphine Requirements, 24 h (mg)	Postoperative Nausea and Vomiting	Pruritus	Hospital Stay Duration (Days)
Risk of Bias	**Very Serious**	**Very Serious**	**Very Serious**	**Serious**	**Very Serious**
Lack of allocation concealment	Some concerns	Some concerns	Some concerns	No	Some concerns
Lack of blinding	Some concerns	Some concerns	Some concerns	No	Some concerns
Incomplete accounting of patients and outcome events	Some concerns	Some concerns	Some concerns	Some concerns	Some concerns
Selective outcome reporting	No	No	No	No	No
Other limitations	No	No	No	No	No

Table 4. *Cont.*

	Pain at Rest, 24 h	Morphine Requirements, 24 h (mg)	Postoperative Nausea and Vomiting	Pruritus	Hospital Stay Duration (Days)
Inconsistency	**Very serious**	**Very serious**	**Serious**	**Not serious**	**Serious**
I^2 (unexplained heterogeneity of results)	Considerable	Considerable	Moderate	None	Considerable
Wide variance of point estimates	No	Yes	Yes	No	Yes
Confidence intervals (CIs) do not overlap	Yes	Yes	No	No	No
Indirectness	**Not serious**	**Not serious**	**Not serious**	**Serious**	**Not serious**
Differences in population	No	No	No	No	No
Differences in interventions	No	No	No	No	No
Differences in outcome measures	No	No	No	Yes	No
Indirect comparisons	No	No	No	No	No
Imprecision	**Not serious**	**Serious**	**Not serious**	**Not serious**	**Not serious**
Few patients	Not serious	Not serious	Not serious	Not serious	Not serious
Wide confidence interval (CI)	Not serious	Serious	Not serious	Not serious	Not serious
Upgrading	**None**	**None**	**None**	**RR < 0.5**	**None**
RR > 2 or RR < 0.5 RR > 5 or RR < 0.2	No	No	No	RR < 0.5	No
Dose-response gradient	No	No	No	No	No
Effect of plausible residual confounding	No	No	No	No	No

4. Discussion

Our meta-analysis revealed positive associations between TENS and various postoperative improvements, including reduced immediate and early postoperative pain, as well as diminished pain at coughing on days 1 and 3. Furthermore, TENS demonstrated effectiveness in decreasing morphine requirements, overall PONV, dizziness, pruritus, and, possibly, hospital length of stay. However, TENS did not show a significant impact on pain during walking. Similarly, sub-analysis based on the type of surgery did not reveal differences in pain scores.

A previously conducted large meta-analysis supports our findings regarding the pain-alleviating effect of TENS. The authors found that TENS reduced acute pain (surgical and non-surgical combined together) by −1.02 [−1.24, −0.79] on a ten-point scale, and postoperative pain by −0.92 [−1.15, −0.69] [27]. All studies combined (92 samples with 4841 participants reporting acute/chronic pain, (non)procedural, etc.) produced similar results: Pain scores in the TENS group were −0.96 [−1.14, −0.78] lower than in the placebo arm [27]. The researchers concluded that while TENS provided analgesic effects, the type of pain, the diagnosis, and the procedure did not affect the impact [27].

Unlike our study, meta-analyses concentrating on specific surgeries observed a statistically significant pain reduction in the TENS group compared to controls. A meta-analysis comprising 559 patients observed lower pain scores on POD one, two, and three in the TENS group compared to the placebo following inguinal hernia repair [24]. In a gynecological study, TENS was found to provide a pain-relieving effect comparable to that of opioids [25]. The use of TENS reduced pain scores at 12, 24, and 48 h following total knee arthroplasty (TKA), according to a meta-analysis of five studies comprising 472 patients [22]. Similarly, TENS reduced pain scores on the first five postoperative days following lung surgeries [23].

Regarding opioid consumption, a meta-analysis of 21 studies found that TENS reduced the postoperative use of opioids by more than 25% [21]. The TENS group consumed fewer opioids in the post-analgesia care unit than the opioid-only group following gynecological surgeries [25]. TENS reduced opioid use at 12, 24, and 48 h following TKA [22]. Similarly, lower pain scores at rest and on coughing were observed in the TENS group after cardiothoracic procedures [26].

Thus, while previous literature demonstrates the pain-relieving and opioid-sparing effects of TENS in the postoperative period following specific surgeries or generally for acute pain management, our study contributes insights to the existing literature on TENS by providing a comprehensive analysis of its effectiveness in postoperative pain management across various surgical contexts. This approach allows for a more generalized evaluation of TENS efficacy in postoperative pain control, offering valuable insights applicable to a wide array of clinical scenarios. Our study examines a comprehensive set of postoperative outcomes, including immediate and early postoperative pain, pain at different time points, pain during specific activities (coughing and walking), as well as morphine requirements, adverse events, and hospital length of stay. This holistic approach provides a more nuanced understanding of TENS's impact on various aspects of postoperative recovery.

This meta-analysis observed a considerable heterogeneity in most outcomes. However, such heterogeneity was anticipated beforehand, given the differences in the durations of interventions, patient characteristics, control groups, surgical procedures, and outcome measures. Variations in TENS protocols, including differences in electrode placement, stimulation parameters, and treatment duration, introduced another source of heterogeneity. Although this heterogeneity posed a challenge in terms of combining and interpreting data, given that the effectiveness of TENS may vary across different contexts, a random effects model was used to account for the between-study variability. Furthermore, subgroup analysis was undertaken wherever possible to obtain more homogeneous results. Sensitivity analyses were also performed to help explore the sources of heterogeneity.

An important limitation of this research was the lack of extended follow-up information, which would have allowed for an assessment of the long-term advantages or potential complications associated with the use of TENS. Furthermore, the quality of the meta-analysis was contingent on the quality of the studies included. As evident from the Cochrane risk of bias, a number of studies had "some concerns" regarding the risk of bias, which subsequently affected the certainty of the evidence. Finally, challenges related to synthesizing data, such as differences in outcome measurement scales or reporting formats, complicated the aggregation of results and the conduct of a comprehensive analysis, as some studies had to be excluded due to these issues.

The implications of our meta-analysis extend both clinically and practically. For clinicians, our findings suggest that incorporating transcutaneous electrical nerve stimulation (TENS) into postoperative pain management protocols can offer tangible benefits, particularly in alleviating early postoperative pain and opioid requirements, and reducing adverse events. This information empowers healthcare providers to make informed decisions about the inclusion of TENS in multimodal analgesia strategies, enhancing overall patient care. Therefore, the study may serve as a guide for clinicians considering TENS as an adjunctive therapy in postoperative care.

From the research point of view, the study identified the need for investigations into the long-term effects of TENS and its impact on specific surgical contexts. Researchers could focus on conducting well-designed, prospective studies with extended follow-up periods to understand the sustained benefits and potential delayed adverse effects of TENS.

5. Conclusions

When considering all types of surgeries, the meta-analysis shows that TENS reduces pain intensity at rest (immediately after surgery and 24 h after surgery), pain intensity during coughing, morphine consumption, the incidence of PONV, and other adverse events, such as PONV, dizziness, and pruritus. We did not find a significant difference between the TENS group and the control group in reducing pain during walking. The subgroup analysis does not show significant differences between the TENS group and controls in pain severity at rest for thoracic, abdominal, or orthopedic surgeries.

Author Contributions: Conceptualization, methodology: D.V.; software: F.N. and Y.G.A.; formal analysis: F.N. and Y.G.A.; writing—original draft preparation: D.V., Y.G.A., N.S., K.T. and M.A.; writing—review and editing: D.V., Y.G.A., M.A., K.T., F.N. and R.T.; quality assessment: M.A., N.S. and K.T. All authors have read and agreed to the published version of the manuscript.

Funding: This work was supported in part by Nazarbayev University Faculty Development Competitive Research grant nos. SOM2021005 (021220FD2851) and 11022021FD2906. The authors have no other relevant affiliations or financial involvement with any organization or entity with a financial interest in or financial conflict with the subject matter or materials discussed in the manuscript apart from those disclosed.

Institutional Review Board Statement: Not applicable.

Informed Consent Statement: Not applicable.

Data Availability Statement: The data can be requested from the corresponding author.

Conflicts of Interest: The authors declare no conflicts of interest.

References

1. Waller-Wise, R. Transcutaneous Electrical Nerve Stimulation: An Overview. *J. Perinat. Educ.* **2022**, *31*, 49–57. [CrossRef] [PubMed]
2. Fiorelli, A.; Morgillo, F.; Milione, R.; Pace, M.C.; Passavanti, M.B.; Laperuta, P.; Aurilio, C.; Santini, M. Control of Post-Thoracotomy Pain by Transcutaneous Electrical Nerve Stimulation: Effect on Serum Cytokine Levels, Visual Analogue Scale, Pulmonary Function and Medication. *Eur. J. Cardio-Thorac. Surg.* **2012**, *41*, 861–868; discussion 868. [CrossRef]
3. Bisgaard, T.; Kehlet, H.; Rosenberg, J. Pain and Convalescence after Laparoscopic Cholecystectomy. *Eur. J. Surg.* **2001**, *167*, 84–96. [CrossRef]
4. Viderman, D.; Aubakirova, M.; Abdildin, Y.G. Transversus Abdominis Plane Block in Colorectal Surgery: A Meta-Analysis. *Front. Med.* **2022**, *8*, 802039. [CrossRef]
5. Viderman, D.; Ben-David, B.; Sarria-Santamera, A. Analysis of bupivacaine and ropivacaine-related cardiac arrests in regional anesthesia: A systematic review of case reports. *Rev. Española Anestesiol. Y Reanim. (Engl. Ed.)* **2021**, *68*, 472–483. [CrossRef]
6. Kim, S.S.; Niu, X.; Elliott, I.A.; Jiang, J.P.; Dann, A.M.; Damato, L.M.; Chung, H.; Girgis, M.D.; King, J.C.; Hines, O.J.; et al. Epidural Analgesia Improves Postoperative Pain Control but Impedes Early Discharge in Patients Undergoing Pancreatic Surgery. *Pancreas* **2019**, *48*, 719–725. [CrossRef] [PubMed]
7. Ben-David, B.; Kaligozhin, Z.; Viderman, D. Quadratus Lumborum Block in Management of Severe Pain after Uterine Artery Embolization. *Eur. J. Pain Lond. Engl.* **2018**, *22*, 1032–1034. [CrossRef] [PubMed]
8. Kikuchi, S.; Kuroda, S.; Nishizaki, M.; Matsusaki, T.; Kuwada, K.; Kimura, Y.; Kagawa, S.; Morimatsu, H.; Fujiwara, T. Comparison of the Effects of Epidural Analgesia and Patient-Controlled Intravenous Analgesia on Postoperative Pain Relief and Recovery after Laparoscopic Gastrectomy for Gastric Cancer. *Surg. Laparosc. Endosc. Percutan. Tech.* **2019**, *29*, 405–408. [CrossRef]
9. Viderman, D.; Dautova, A.; Sarria-Santamera, A. Erector Spinae Plane Block in Acute Interventional Pain Management: A Systematic Review. *Scand. J. Pain* **2021**, *21*, 671–679. [CrossRef]
10. Viderman, D.; Aubakirova, M.; Umbetzhanov, Y.; Kulkaeva, G.; Shalekenov, S.B.; Abdildin, Y.G. Ultrasound-guided erector spinae plane block in thoracolumbar spinal surgery: A systematic review and meta-analysis. *Front. Med.* **2022**, *9*, 932101. [CrossRef]
11. Abdildin, Y.; Tapinova, K.; Nugumanova, M.; Viderman, D. Transversus Abdominis Plane Block in Adult Open Liver Surgery Patients: A Systematic Review with Meta-Analysis of Randomized Controlled Trials. *J. Visc. Surg.* **2023**, *160*, 253–260. [CrossRef] [PubMed]
12. Chou, R.; Gordon, D.B.; De Leon-Casasola, O.A.; Rosenberg, J.M.; Bickler, S.; Brennan, T.; Carter, T.; Cassidy, C.L.; Chittenden, E.H.; Degenhardt, E.; et al. Management of Postoperative Pain: A Clinical Practice Guideline from the American Pain Society,

the American Society of Regional Anesthesia and Pain Medicine, and the American Society of Anesthesiologists' Committee on Regional Anesthesia, Executive Committee, and Administrative Council. *J. Pain* **2016**, *17*, 131–157. [CrossRef] [PubMed]

13. Silva, M.B.; de Melo, P.R.; de Oliveira, N.M.L.; Crema, E.; Fernandes, L.F.R.M. Analgesic Effect of Transcutaneous Electrical Nerve Stimulation after Laparoscopic Cholecystectomy. *Am. J. Phys. Med. Rehabil.* **2012**, *91*, 652–657. [CrossRef] [PubMed]
14. Tokuda, M.; Tabira, K.; Masuda, T.; Nishiwada, T.; Shomoto, K. Effect of Modulated-Frequency and Modulated-Intensity Transcutaneous Electrical Nerve Stimulation after Abdominal Surgery: A Randomized Controlled Trial. *Clin. J. Pain* **2014**, *30*, 565–570. [CrossRef] [PubMed]
15. Borges, M.R.; de Oliveira, N.M.L.; Antonelli, I.B.S.; Silva, M.B.; Crema, E.; Fernandes, L.F.R.M. Transcutaneous Electrical Nerve Stimulation Is Superior than Placebo and Control for Postoperative Pain Relief. *Pain Manag.* **2020**, *10*, 235–246. [CrossRef] [PubMed]
16. Mannheimer, J.S.; Lampe, G.N. *Clinical Transcutaneous Electrical Nerve Stimulation*; F A Davis Company: Philadelphia, PA, USA, 1984.
17. Sluka, K.A.; Walsh, D. Transcutaneous Electrical Nerve Stimulation: Basic Science Mechanisms and Clinical Effectiveness. *J. Pain* **2003**, *4*, 109–121. [CrossRef] [PubMed]
18. Woolf, C.J.; Mitchell, D.; Barrett, G.D. Antinociceptive Effect of Peripheral Segmental Electrical Stimulation in the Rat. *Pain* **1980**, *8*, 237–252. [CrossRef]
19. Melzack, R.; Wall, P.D. Pain Mechanisms: A New Theory. *Science* **1965**, *150*, 971–979. [CrossRef]
20. Kalra, A.; Urban, M.O.; Sluka, K.A. Blockade of Opioid Receptors in Rostral Ventral Medulla Prevents Antihyperalgesia Produced by Transcutaneous Electrical Nerve Stimulation (TENS). *J. Pharmacol. Exp. Ther.* **2001**, *298*, 257–263.
21. Bjordal, J.M.; Johnson, M.I.; Ljunggreen, A.E. Transcutaneous Electrical Nerve Stimulation (TENS) Can Reduce Postoperative Analgesic Consumption. A Meta-Analysis with Assessment of Optimal Treatment Parameters for Postoperative Pain. *Eur. J. Pain Lond. Engl.* **2003**, *7*, 181–188. [CrossRef]
22. Li, J.; Song, Y. Transcutaneous Electrical Nerve Stimulation for Postoperative Pain Control after Total Knee Arthroplasty: A Meta-Analysis of Randomized Controlled Trials. *Medicine* **2017**, *96*, e8036. [CrossRef] [PubMed]
23. Zhou, J.; Dan, Y.; Yixian, Y.; Lyu, M.; Zhong, J.; Wang, Z.; Zhu, Y.; Liu, L. Efficacy of Transcutaneous Electronic Nerve Stimulation in Postoperative Analgesia after Pulmonary Surgery: A Systematic Review and Meta-Analysis. *Am. J. Phys. Med. Rehabil.* **2020**, *99*, 241–249. [CrossRef] [PubMed]
24. Watanabe, J.; Izumi, N.; Kobayashi, F.; Miki, A.; Sata, N. Efficacy and Safety of Transcutaneous Electrical Nerve Stimulation in Patients Undergoing Inguinal Hernia Repair: A Systematic Review and Meta-Analysis. *JMA J.* **2023**, *6*, 371–380. [CrossRef] [PubMed]
25. Piasecki, A.; Ögren, C.; Thörn, S.-E.; Olausson, A.; Svensson, C.J.; Platon, B.; Wolf, A.; Andréll, P. High-Frequency, High-Intensity Transcutaneous Electrical Nerve Stimulation Compared with Opioids for Pain Relief after Gynecological Surgery: A Systematic Review and Meta-Analysis. *Scand. J. Pain* **2023**, *24*, 20230068. [CrossRef]
26. Cardinali, A.; Celini, D.; Chaplik, M.; Grasso, E.; Nemec, E.C. Efficacy of Transcutaneous Electrical Nerve Stimulation for Postoperative Pain, Pulmonary Function, and Opioid Consumption Following Cardiothoracic Procedures: A Systematic Review. *Neuromod. Technol. Neural Interface* **2021**, *24*, 1439–1450. [CrossRef]
27. Johnson, M.I.; Paley, C.A.; Jones, G.; Mulvey, M.R.; Wittkopf, P.G. Efficacy and Safety of Transcutaneous Electrical Nerve Stimulation (TENS) for Acute and Chronic Pain in Adults: A Systematic Review and Meta-Analysis of 381 Studies (the Meta-TENS Study). *BMJ Open* **2022**, *12*, e051073. [CrossRef]
28. Page, M.J.; McKenzie, J.E.; Bossuyt, P.M.; Boutron, I.; Hoffmann, T.C.; Mulrow, C.D.; Shamseer, L.; Tetzlaff, J.M.; Akl, E.A.; Brennan, S.E.; et al. The PRISMA 2020 Statement: An Updated Guideline for Reporting Systematic Reviews. *BMJ* **2021**, *372*, n71. [CrossRef] [PubMed]
29. Higgins, J.P.T.; Thomas, J.; Chandler, J.; Cumpston, M.; Li, T.; Page, M.J.; Welch, V.A. (Eds.) *Cochrane Handbook for Systematic Reviews of Interventions*; Version 6.4 (Updated August 2023); Cochrane: London, UK, 2023; Available online: www.training. cochrane.org/handbook (accessed on 1 December 2022).
30. Luo, D.; Wan, X.; Liu, J.; Tong, T. Optimally Estimating the Sample Mean from the Sample Size, Median, Mid-Range, and/or Mid-Quartile Range. *Stat. Methods Med. Res.* **2018**, *27*, 1785–1805. [CrossRef]
31. Wan, X.; Wang, W.; Liu, J.; Tong, T. Estimating the Sample Mean and Standard Deviation from the Sample Size, Median, Range and/or Interquartile Range. *BMC Med. Res. Methodol.* **2014**, *14*, 135. [CrossRef]
32. Sterne, J.A.C.; Savović, J.; Page, M.J.; Elbers, R.G.; Blencowe, N.S.; Boutron, I.; Cates, C.J.; Cheng, H.-Y.; Corbett, M.S.; Eldridge, S.M.; et al. RoB 2: A Revised Tool for Assessing Risk of Bias in Randomised Trials. *BMJ* **2019**, *366*, l4898. [CrossRef]
33. Guyatt, G.H.; Oxman, A.D.; Schünemann, H.J.; Tugwell, P.; Knottnerus, A. GRADE Guidelines: A New Series of Articles in the Journal of Clinical Epidemiology. *J. Clin. Epidemiol.* **2011**, *64*, 380–382. [CrossRef] [PubMed]
34. Ilfeld, B.M.; Plunkett, A.; Vijjeswarapu, A.M.; Hackworth, R.; Dhanjal, S.; Turan, A.; Cohen, S.P.; Eisenach, J.C.; Griffith, S.; Hanling, S.; et al. Percutaneous Peripheral Nerve Stimulation (Neuromodulation) for Postoperative Pain: A Randomized, Sham-Controlled Pilot Study. *Anesthesiology* **2021**, *135*, 95–110. [CrossRef] [PubMed]
35. da Silva, M.P.; Liebano, R.E.; Rodrigues, V.A.; Abla, L.E.F.; Ferreira, L.M. Transcutaneous Electrical Nerve Stimulation for Pain Relief after Liposuction: A Randomized Controlled Trial. *Aesthetic Plast. Surg.* **2015**, *39*, 262–269. [CrossRef] [PubMed]

36. Erden, S.; Senol Celik, S. The Effect of Transcutaneous Electrical Nerve Stimulation on Post-Thoracotomy Pain. *Contemp. Nurse* **2015**, *51*, 163–170. [CrossRef] [PubMed]
37. Asgari, Z.; Tavoli, Z.; Hosseini, R.; Nataj, M.; Tabatabaei, F.; Dehghanizadeh, F.; Haji-Amoo-Assar, H.; Sepidarkish, M.; Montazeri, A. A Comparative Study between Transcutaneous Electrical Nerve Stimulation and Fentanyl to Relieve Shoulder Pain during Laparoscopic Gynecologic Surgery under Spinal Anesthesia: A Randomized Clinical Trail. *Pain Res. Manag.* **2018**, *2018*, 9715142. [CrossRef] [PubMed]
38. Bjerså, K.; Jildenstaal, P.; Jakobsson, J.; Egardt, M.; Fagevik Olsén, M. Adjunct High Frequency Transcutaneous Electric Stimulation (TENS) for Postoperative Pain Management during Weaning from Epidural Analgesia Following Colon Surgery: Results from a Controlled Pilot Study. *Pain Manag. Nurs. Off. J. Am. Soc. Pain Manag. Nurses* **2015**, *16*, 944–950. [CrossRef] [PubMed]
39. Lima, P.M.B.; de Brito Farias, R.T.F.; Carvalho, A.C.A.; da Silva, P.N.C.; Ferraz Filho, N.A.; de Brito, R.F. Estimulação elétrica nervosa transcutânea após cirurgia de revascularização miocárdica. *Braz. J. Cardiovasc. Surg.* **2011**, *26*, 591–596. [CrossRef]
40. Ferreira, F.C.; Issy, A.M.; Sakata, R.K. Assessing the Effects of Transcutaneous Electrical Nerve Stimulation (TENS) in Post-Thoracotomy Analgesia. *Rev. Bras. Anestesiol.* **2011**, *61*, 561–567. [CrossRef]
41. Beckwée, D.; Bautmans, I.; Lefeber, N.; Lievens, P.; Scheerlinck, T.; Vaes, P. Effect of Transcutaneous Electric Nerve Stimulation on Pain after Total Knee Arthroplasty: A Blind Randomized Controlled Trial. *J. Knee Surg.* **2018**, *31*, 189–196. [CrossRef]
42. Chiu, J.H.; Chen, W.S.; Chen, C.H.; Jiang, J.K.; Tang, G.J.; Lui, W.Y.; Lin, J.K. Effect of Transcutaneous Electrical Nerve Stimulation for Pain Relief on Patients Undergoing Hemorrhoidectomy: Prospective, Randomized, Controlled Trial. *Dis. Colon Rectum* **1999**, *42*, 180–185. [CrossRef]
43. Elboim-Gabyzon, M.; Andrawus Najjar, S.; Shtarker, H. Effects of Transcutaneous Electrical Nerve Stimulation (TENS) on Acute Postoperative Pain Intensity and Mobility after Hip Fracture: A Double-Blinded, Randomized Trial. *Clin. Interv. Aging* **2019**, *14*, 1841–1850. [CrossRef] [PubMed]
44. Engen, D.J.; Carns, P.E.; Allen, M.S.; Bauer, B.A.; Loehrer, L.L.; Cha, S.S.; Chartrand, C.M.; Eggler, E.J.; Cutshall, S.M.; Wahner-Roedler, D.L. Evaluating Efficacy and Feasibility of Transcutaneous Electrical Nerve Stimulation for Postoperative Pain after Video-Assisted Thoracoscopic Surgery: A Randomized Pilot Trial. *Complement. Ther. Clin. Pract.* **2016**, *23*, 141–148. [CrossRef] [PubMed]
45. Erden, S.; Yurtseven, Ş.; Demir, S.G.; Arslan, S.; Arslan, U.E.; Dalcı, K. Effects of Transcutaneous Electrical Nerve Stimulation on Mastectomy Pain, Patient Satisfaction, and Patient Outcomes. *J. Perianesthesia Nurs.* **2022**, *37*, 485–492. [CrossRef] [PubMed]
46. Erdogan, M.; Erdogan, A.; Erbil, N.; Karakaya, H.K.; Demircan, A. Prospective, Randomized, Placebo-Controlled Study of the Effect of TENS on Postthoracotomy Pain and Pulmonary Function. *World J. Surg.* **2005**, *29*, 1563–1570. [CrossRef] [PubMed]
47. Kurata, N.B.; Ghatnekar, R.J.; Mercer, E.; Chin, J.M.; Kaneshiro, B.; Yamasato, K.S. Transcutaneous Electrical Nerve Stimulation for Post-Cesarean Birth Pain Control: A Randomized Controlled Trial. *Obstet. Gynecol.* **2022**, *140*, 174–180. [CrossRef] [PubMed]
48. Kara, B.; Baskurt, F.; Acar, S.; Karadibak, D.; Ciftci, L.; Erbayraktar, S.; Gokmen, A.N. The Effect of TENS on Pain, Function, Depression, and Analgesic Consumption in the Early Postoperative Period with Spinal Surgery Patients. *Turk. Neurosurg.* **2011**, *21*, 618–624. [CrossRef] [PubMed]
49. Parseliunas, A.; Paskauskas, S.; Kubiliute, E.; Vaitekunas, J.; Venskutonis, D. Transcutaneous Electric Nerve Stimulation Reduces Acute Postoperative Pain and Analgesic Use after Open Inguinal Hernia Surgery: A Randomized, Double-Blind, Placebo-Controlled Trial. *J. Pain* **2021**, *22*, 533–544. [CrossRef]
50. Sezen, C.B.; Akboga, S.A.; Celik, A.; Kalafat, C.E.; Tastepe, A.I. Transcutaneous Electrical Nerve Stimulation Effect on Postoperative Complications. *Asian Cardiovasc. Thorac. Ann.* **2017**, *25*, 276–280. [CrossRef]
51. Smedley, F.; Taube, M.; Wastell, C. Transcutaneous Electrical Nerve Stimulation for Pain Relief Following Inguinal Hernia Repair: A Controlled Trial. *Eur. Surg. Res.* **1988**, *20*, 233–237. [CrossRef]
52. Yu, X.; Zhang, F.; Chen, B. The Effect of TEAS on the Quality of Early Recovery in Patients Undergoing Gynecological Laparoscopic Surgery: A Prospective, Randomized, Placebo-Controlled Trial. *Trials* **2020**, *21*, 43. [CrossRef]
53. Zhang, C.; Xiao, Z.; Zhang, X.; Guo, L.; Sun, W.; Tai, C.; Jiang, Z.; Liu, Y. Transcutaneous Electrical Stimulation of Somatic Afferent Nerves in the Foot Relieved Symptoms Related to Postoperative Bladder Spasms. *BMC Urol.* **2017**, *17*, 58. [CrossRef] [PubMed]
54. Zhang, B.; Xu, F.; Hu, P.; Zhang, M.; Tong, K.; Ma, G.; Xu, Y.; Zhu, L.; Chen, J.D.Z. Needleless Transcutaneous Electrical Acustimulation: A Pilot Study Evaluating Improvement in Post-Operative Recovery. *Am. J. Gastroenterol.* **2018**, *113*, 1026–1035. [CrossRef] [PubMed]
55. Chen, W.; Liu, C.; Yang, Y.; Tian, L. The Effect of Transcutaneous Electrical Nerve Stimulation (TENS) on Pain Control and Phenylethanolamine-N-Methyltransferase (PNMT) Gene Expression after Cesarean Section. *Cell. Mol. Biol.* **2021**, *67*, 153–157. [CrossRef] [PubMed]
56. Forogh, B.; Aslanpour, H.; Fallah, E.; Babaei-Ghazani, A.; Ebadi, S. Adding High-Frequency Transcutaneous Electrical Nerve Stimulation to the First Phase of Post Anterior Cruciate Ligament Reconstruction Rehabilitation Does Not Improve Pain and Function in Young Male Athletes More than Exercise Alone: A Randomized Single-Blind Clinical Trial. *Disabil. Rehabil.* **2019**, *41*, 514–522. [CrossRef] [PubMed]
57. Galli, T.T.; Chiavegato, L.D.; Liebano, R.E. Effects of TENS in Living Kidney Donors Submitted to Open Nephrectomy: A Randomized Placebo-Controlled Trial. *Eur. J. Pain Lond. Engl.* **2015**, *19*, 67–76. [CrossRef]
58. Gregorini, C.; Cipriano Junior, G.; de Aquino, L.M.; Branco, J.N.R.; Bernardelli, G.F. Short-Duration Transcutaneous Electrical Nerve Stimulation in the Postoperative Period of Cardiac Surgery. *Arq. Bras. Cardiol.* **2010**, *94*, 325–331. [CrossRef]

59. Mahure, S.A.; Rokito, A.S.; Kwon, Y.W. Transcutaneous Electrical Nerve Stimulation for Postoperative Pain Relief after Arthroscopic Rotator Cuff Repair: A Prospective Double-Blinded Randomized Trial. *J. Shoulder Elbow Surg.* **2017**, *26*, 1508–1513. [CrossRef]

60. Rakel, B.; Frantz, R. Effectiveness of Transcutaneous Electrical Nerve Stimulation on Postoperative Pain with Movement. *J. Pain* **2003**, *4*, 455–464. [CrossRef]

61. Jahangirifard, A.; Razavi, M.; Ahmadi, Z.H.; Forozeshfard, M. Effect of TENS on Postoperative Pain and Pulmonary Function in Patients Undergoing Coronary Artery Bypass Surgery. *Pain Manag. Nurs.* **2018**, *19*, 408–414. [CrossRef]

62. Bjerså, K.; Andersson, T. High Frequency TENS as a Complement for Pain Relief in Postoperative Transition from Epidural to General Analgesia after Pancreatic Resection. *Complement. Ther. Clin. Pract.* **2014**, *20*, 5–10. [CrossRef]

63. Cuschieri, R.J.; Morran, C.G.; McArdle, C.S. Transcutaneous Electrical Stimulation for Postoperative Pain. *Ann. R. Coll. Surg. Engl.* **1985**, *67*, 127–129. [PubMed]

64. McCallum, M.I.; Glynn, C.J.; Moore, R.A.; Lammer, P.; Phillips, A.M. Transcutaneous Electrical Nerve Stimulation in the Management of Acute Postoperative Pain. *Br. J. Anaesth.* **1988**, *61*, 308–312. [CrossRef] [PubMed]

65. Navarathnam, R.G.; Wang, I.Y.; Thomas, D.; Klineberg, P.L. Evaluation of the Transcutaneous Electrical Nerve Stimulator for Postoperative Analgesia Following Cardiac Surgery. *Anaesth. Intensive Care* **1984**, *12*, 345–350. [CrossRef] [PubMed]

66. Benedetti, F.; Amanzio, M.; Casadio, C.; Cavallo, A.; Cianci, R.; Giobbe, R.; Mancuso, M.; Ruffini, E.; Maggi, G. Control of Postoperative Pain by Transcutaneous Electrical Nerve Stimulation after Thoracic Operations. *Ann. Thorac. Surg.* **1997**, *63*, 773–776. [CrossRef] [PubMed]

67. Hamza, M.A.; White, P.F.; Ahmed, H.E.; Ghoname, E.A. Effect of the Frequency of Transcutaneous Electrical Nerve Stimulation on the Postoperative Opioid Analgesic Requirement and Recovery Profile. *Anesthesiology* **1999**, *91*, 1232–1238. [CrossRef] [PubMed]

68. Laitinen, J.; Nuutinen, L. Failure of Transcutaneous Electrical Nerve Stimulation and Indomethacin to Reduce Opiate Requirement Following Cholecystectomy. *Acta Anaesthesiol. Scand.* **1991**, *35*, 700–705. [CrossRef]

69. Solak, O.; Turna, A.; Pekcolaklar, A.; Metin, M.; Sayar, A.; Solak, O.; Gürses, A. Transcutaneous Electric Nerve Stimulation for the Treatment of Postthoracotomy Pain: A Randomized Prospective Study. *Thorac. Cardiovasc. Surg.* **2007**, *55*, 182–185. [CrossRef]

70. Stubbing, J.F.; Jellicoe, J.A. Transcutaneous Electrical Nerve Stimulation after Thoracotomy. Pain Relief and Peak Expiratory Flow Rate—A Trial of Transcutaneous Electrical Nerve Stimulation. *Anaesthesia* **1988**, *43*, 296–298. [CrossRef]

71. Wang, H.; Xie, Y.; Zhang, Q.; Xu, N.; Zhong, H.; Dong, H.; Liu, L.; Jiang, T.; Wang, Q.; Xiong, L. Transcutaneous Electric Acupoint Stimulation Reduces Intra-Operative Remifentanil Consumption and Alleviates Postoperative Side-Effects in Patients Undergoing Sinusotomy: A Prospective, Randomized, Placebo-Controlled Trial. *Br. J. Anaesth.* **2014**, *112*, 1075–1082. [CrossRef]

72. Platon, B.; Andréll, P.; Raner, C.; Rudolph, M.; Dvoretsky, A.; Mannheimer, C. High-Frequency, High-Intensity Transcutaneous Electrical Nerve Stimulation as Treatment of Pain after Surgical Abortion. *Pain* **2010**, *148*, 114–119. [CrossRef]

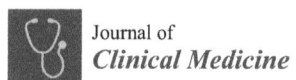

Journal of
Clinical Medicine

Article

Ultrasound Guided Parasternal Block for Perioperative Analgesia in Cardiac Surgery: A Prospective Study

Giuseppe Pascarella [1], Fabio Costa [1], Giulia Nonnis [2], Alessandro Strumia [1,*], Domenico Sarubbi [1], Lorenzo Schiavoni [1], Annalaura Di Pumpo [1], Lara Mortini [1], Stefania Grande [1], Andrea Attanasio [3], Giovanni Gadotti [4], Alessandro De Cassai [5], Alessia Mattei [1], Antonio Nenna [6], Massimo Chello [6], Rita Cataldo [1], Felice Eugenio Agrò [1] and Massimiliano Carassiti [1]

1   Unit of Anaesthesia and Intensive Care, Fondazione Policlinico Universitario Campus Bio-Medico, 00128 Rome, Italy
2   Unit of Anaesthesia and Intensive Care, Ospedale dei Castelli, Ariccia, 00040 Rome, Italy
3   Unit of Anaesthesia and Intensive Care, Ospedale Sant Orsola, 40138 Bologna, Italy
4   Unit of Anaesthesia and Intensive Care, Azienda Ospedaliera San Camillo Forlanini, 00152 Rome, Italy
5   Unit of Anaesthesia and Intensive Care, University Hospital of Padua, 35128 Padua, Italy
6   Unit of Cardiac Surgery, Fondazione Policlinico Universitario Campus Bio-Medico, 00128 Rome, Italy
*   Correspondence: a.strumia@policlinicocampus.it; Tel.: +39-3471403574

Abstract: Ultrasound guided parasternal block is a regional anaesthesia technique targeting the anterior branches of intercostal nerves, which supply the anterior thoracic wall. The aim of this prospective study is to assess the efficacy of parasternal block to manage postoperative analgesia and reduce opioid consumption in patients undergoing cardiac surgery throughout sternotomy. A total of 126 consecutive patients were allocated to two different groups, receiving (Parasternal group) or not (Control group) preoperative ultrasound guided bilateral parasternal block with 20 mL of 0.5% ropivacaine per side. The following data were recorded: postoperative pain expressed by a 0–10 numeric rating scale (NRS), intraoperative fentanyl consumption, postoperative morphine consumption, time to extubation and perioperative pulmonary performance at incentive spirometry. Postoperative NRS was not significantly different between Parasternal and Control groups with a median (IQR) of 2 (0–4.5) vs. 3 (0–6) upon awakening ($p = 0.07$); 0 (0–3) vs. 2 (0–4) at 6 h ($p = 0.46$); 0 (0–2) vs. 0 (0–2) at 12 h ($p = 0.57$). Postoperative morphine consumption was similar among groups. However, intraoperative fentanyl consumption was significantly lower in the Parasternal group [406.3 ± 81.6 mcg vs. 864.3 ± 154.4, ($p < 0.001$)]. Parasternal group showed shorter times to extubation [(191 ± 58 min vs. 305 ± 72 min, (p)] and better performance at incentive spirometer with a median (IQR) of 2 raised balls (1–2) vs. 1 (1–2) after awakening ($p = 0.04$). Ultrasound guided parasternal block provided an optimal perioperative analgesia with a significant reduction in intraoperative opioid consumption, time to extubation and a better postoperative performance at spirometry when compared to the Control group.

Keywords: parasternal block; regional anaesthesia; cardiac surgery; cardiac anaesthesia; pain management

Citation: Pascarella, G.; Costa, F.; Nonnis, G.; Strumia, A.; Sarubbi, D.; Schiavoni, L.; Di Pumpo, A.; Mortini, L.; Grande, S.; Attanasio, A.; et al. Ultrasound Guided Parasternal Block for Perioperative Analgesia in Cardiac Surgery: A Prospective Study. *J. Clin. Med.* **2023**, *12*, 2060. https://doi.org/10.3390/jcm12052060

Academic Editor: Chun Yang and Young-Tae Jeon

Received: 2 January 2023
Revised: 3 February 2023
Accepted: 2 March 2023
Published: 6 March 2023

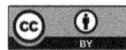
1. Introduction

Due to the improvement in life expectancy, heart surgery has become increasingly common among elderly population. However, due to the frailty and comorbidities of these patients, perioperative complications are frequent. Moreover, the impact of anaesthetics and analgesic drugs play an important role on the perioperative course [1].

Post-operative pain is mainly related to median surgical sternotomy; it is intense and difficult to control, especially in the immediate few hours after surgery [2]. It requires high doses of opiates that may lead to different side effects, such as nausea, vomiting, respiratory issues and postoperative delirium. Furthermore, high anaesthetic drug administration can cause a delay in extubating time and weaning from mechanical ventilation. Moreover, sympathetic stimulus and chest pain may induce an important reduction in thoracic excursion, finally facilitating pulmonary infections [3].

Recently, many thoracic fascial plane blocks have been proven to be a valid option in controlling pain in cardiac, thoracic and breast surgery [4–7].

The sternal region is innervated by the anterior branches of intercostal nerves, which arise from the anterior branches of the spinal nerves from T1 to T11 [8]. Parasternal block is a recent block which targets these branches due to the injection of local anaesthetic between the pectoral major and the intercostal muscles, proximal to the sternum. To obtain a good analgesic cover, the block needs to be performed bilaterally with a spread from the II to the VI intercostal spaces.

Several studies have investigated the parasternal block in cardiac patients trying to understand its impact on intra- and post- operative pain [9–13]; however, most of the studies are retrospective or based on a small number of patients.

The aim of this prospective study is to assess the efficacy of parasternal block to manage postoperative analgesia, reduce opioid consumption and improve respiratory function in patients undergoing cardiac surgery.

2. Materials and Methods

This study was approved by Campus BioMedico Hospital Ethical Committee (protocol number 20/20 PAR ComEt CBM) and was registered on clinicaltrias.gov (NCT04319588).

A total of 126 patients who underwent elective cardiac surgery were enrolled between November 2019 and March 2020. Written informed consent was obtained from all the subjects. Inclusion criteria to participate included: patients aged 18 years or older, ASA physical status I-IV and candidates for elective cardiac surgery with median sternotomy. Exclusion criteria included: allergy to local anaesthetics, site of puncture infection, weight < 30 Kg, impaired cerebral function and patient's disapproval.

All patients received general anaesthesia conducted with sevoflurane 2%, fentanyl 3–5 mcg/kg, remifentanil continuous infusion 0.1 mcg/kg/min (depending on clinical judgment of the anaesthetist), rocuronium 0.8–1 mg/kg and propofol 2% continuous infusion (in patients who underwent extracorporeal circulation). The administration of adjunctive boluses of fentanyl (1 mcg/kg) intraoperatively was decided by the anaesthetists based on the hemodynamic parameter variations suggesting pain, such as a rapid increase in blood pressure and heart rate in the absence of fluid loading or amine infusion.

Patients were freely allocated in two groups:

- The *"Parasternal"* group received ultrasound guided bilateral parasternal block after general anaesthesia induction and an infiltration with local anaesthetic of the surgical drainage sites at the end of surgery.
- The *"Control"* group received just the infiltration with local anaesthetic of the surgical drainage sites at the end of surgery.

Drainages sites' infiltration was provided since the parasternal block does not target the sub-phrenic area where the drainages exit the skin. Moreover, we performed it in both groups to eliminate potential bias generated by patients' upper abdominal pain perception.

Both groups received the same protocol of multimodal perioperative analgesia, which included: dexamethasone 0.1 mg/kg i.v. intraoperative; ketorolac 60 mg/24 h i.v. and paracetamol 1 g every 8 h i.v., postoperatively. In addition, morphine 2 mg i.v. was administered in the case of postoperative NRS pain scores $\geq$ 6.

A spirometry evaluation was performed both immediately before surgery and in the postoperative period with the aim to evaluate respiratory function after the surgical intervention and to compare to baseline values. This evaluation was performed with the TriFlo Inspiratory Exerciser®, a device which consist of three air columns with different weights and coloured balls that move up when the patient inhales.

At the end of the operation, all patients were transferred to the intensive care unit (ICU) for weaning from invasive mechanical ventilation and immediate postoperative monitoring.

Data collected: anthropometric data; chronic opiate medications; diabetes mellitus; pre-existing pulmonary conditions; type of surgery—aortocoronary bypass, off pump aortocoronary bypass, valvular surgery and ascending aortic surgery; length of surgery; postoperative pain at extubation and after 6–12–24 h on a 0–10 numeric rating scale (NRS) expressed as maximum pain experienced during that period of time; postoperative opiates consumption: time to first morphine bolus administration (from the patient awakening); total morphine consumption during the first 24 h after surgery; intraoperative opiate consumption (fentanyl, remifentanil); time to extubation; side effects—nausea and vomiting; delirium (using the Mini Mental State Examination); and respiratory performance with the TriFlo expressed as the number of balls moved up before and after the surgery. All the data in the ICU (e.g., NRS, postoperative consumption, pulmonary function, etc.) were collected by the ICU nurses specialized in the management of cardiac surgery patients.

2.1. Block Execution

The patients in the Parasternal group received bilateral ultrasound guided parasternal block immediately after induction of general anaesthesia and intubation [14]. The block was executed with aseptic technique right after patient intubation and before surgical incision. A high-frequency ultrasound probe was positioned immediately lateral to the sternum, identifying the second and the fourth intercostal spaces (Figure 1A). Then, an echogenic 100 mm needle (Stimuplex ultra 360, BBraun Deutschland GmbH & Co., Melsugen, Germany) was advanced through the skin with an in-plane approach and an injection of 10 mL 0.5% ropivacaine was performed between pectoral major and intercostal muscles, bilaterally, with a total dose of 200 mg of ropivacaine (Figure 1B). Success of the block was confirmed by the presence of the double hypoechogenic V sign indicative of correct presence of local anaesthetic between the two muscular fasciae [15]. All the blocks were performed by two expert anaesthesiologists in regional anaesthesia who had already performed more than 50 parasternal blocks before enrolling the first patient.

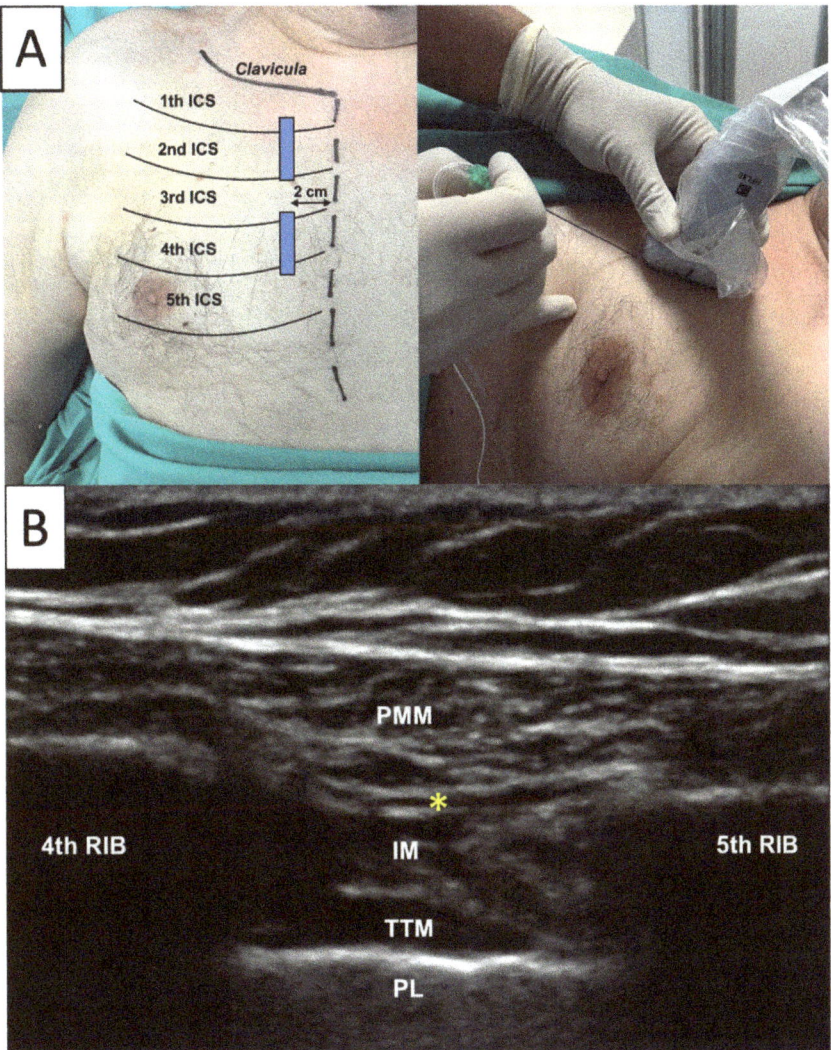

Figure 1. Parasternal Block Execution. *Legend:* A high frequency ultrasound probe was positioned immediately lateral to the sternum identifying the second and the fourth intercostal spaces (**A**). Then, an echogenic 100 mm needle (Stimuplex ultra-360, BBraun Deutschland GmbH & Co., Melsugen, Germany) was advanced through the skin with an in-plane approach and an injection of 10 mL 0.5% ropivacaine was performed between pectoral major and intercostal muscles for every intercostal space, bilaterally, with a total dose of 200 mg of ropivacaine (**B**). PMM: pectoral major muscle; IM: intercostal muscles; TTM: transversus thoracis muscle; PL: pleura; *: point of injection.

At the end of the surgery, both groups received a local infiltration of the surgical drainages with ropivacaine 0.25% 20 mL performed by the surgeon.

2.2. Statistical Analysis

To calculate a sample size, we focused on our primary hypothesis that perioperative analgesia is improved with the parasternal block. We estimated the density of pain scores (mean 2; SD 1.5) based on published data regarding the use of parasternal block for cardiac surgery [16]. To simulate power, we used the truncated Gaussian distribution with range

0–10; standard deviation = 1.5; PARASTERNAL group mean = 2. Under these assumptions and 2-sided α = 5%, we simulated 10,000 trials with sample size of 63 per group. With an overall sample size of 126 subjects, we have at least 90% power to detect group differences in pain as small as approximately 1.

Statistical analysis and graphical presentation were obtained thanks to the use of the GraphPad Prism 8 software (GraphPad Software Inc., San Diego, CA, USA).

The values of continuous quantitative variables are expressed as mean ± standard deviation (SD); the values of discrete variables are expressed as median and interquartile range (IQR). Qualitative variables are expressed as number of observations and percentage of distribution.

The parametric distribution of numerical variables was evaluated using the Shapiro–Wilk normality test. Difference between groups was assessed by T-Student test for continuous parametric variables, while Wilcoxon–Mann–Whitney U test was used when appropriate. Bonferroni–Dunn correction has been applied to multiple repeated measures in order to reduce the risk of type 1 error.

Categorical variables were compared with Pearson's χ^2 test. The level of statistical significance was set for p value < 0.05.

3. Results

A total of 126 patients were enrolled in this study. In the Parasternal group, the median age was 67 ± 10 years, while in the Control group was 70 ± 10; both groups had a higher prevalence of males, and the mean body mass index (BMI) was 26.5 kg/m^2 ± 2.1 in the Parasternal group and 27.8 kg/m^2 ± 1.1 in the Control group.

Aortocoronary bypass in extracorporeal circulation (CEC) was the most performed intervention overall (57% in Parasternal group and 65% in Control group), followed by valvular surgery (30% and 25%, respectively); less frequent were off-pump aortocoronary bypasses, combined bypasses plus valvular surgery and thoracic aorta aneurysm. Surgical average duration was 230.7 ± 53.5 min in the Parasternal group, and 213 ± 40.8 min in the Control group (Table 1).

Table 1. Patients' characteristics.

	Parasternal (63)	Control (63)	p-Value
Age (years)	67 ± 10	69.6 ± 10	0.17
Sex (M/F)	33/30	35/28	0.8
BMI (kg/m^2)	26.7 ± 4	26.5 ± 3.3	0.9
Chronic opiates medication	2 (3%)	3 (5%)	>0.9
Diabetes Mellitus	13 (21%)	12(19%)	>0.9
Pre-existing pulmonary disorders	11 (17%)	10 (16%)	0.88
Type of surgery			
CABG	36 (57%)	41 (65%)	
CABG off pump	3 (5%)	4 (6%)	
Valvular surgery	19 (30%)	16 (25%)	0.6
CABG + valvular surgery	4 (6%)	1 (2%)	
Thoracic aorta aneurysm	1 (2%)	1 (2%)	
Surgery duration (min)	230.7 ± 53.5	213 ± 40.8	0.08

Values are expressed in mean ± standard deviation or in number of patients (%); CABG = coronary artery bypass surgery.

Intraoperative fentanyl consumption emerged to be significantly higher in the Control group with a mean of 864.3 mcg compared to 406.3 mcg in the Parasternal group (p-value < 0.001). Intraoperative remifentanil administration was not statistically significative between the two groups.

Median (IQR) postoperative pain at awakening, expressed as maximum NRS scale value (range 0–10), was 2 (0–4.5) in the Parasternal and 3 (0–6) in the Control group (p = 0.07); in the next 6 h it was 0 (0–3) in the Parasternal and 2 (0–4) in the Control group, while it was 0 in both groups during the following hours. However, pain was always under 4 at 48 h after extubation (mild pain) in both groups.

Postoperative opiates were requested by 30% of patients in the Parasternal group and by 29% of patients in the Control group. Furthermore, both groups showed no difference in the median (IQR) consumption of postoperative morphine during the first 24 h (0 (0–2) mg). Furthermore, the median (IQR) time to first opioid administration was similar (30 (10–45) mg for parasternal group vs. 30 (11–60) mg for control group) (Table 2).

Table 2. Main Outcomes.

	Parasternal	Control	*p*-Value
Intraoperative fentanyl (γ)	406.3 ± 81.6	864.3 ± 154.4	**<0.001**
Intraoperative remifentanil (γ)	336.1 ± 13.1	338.3 ± 13.5	0.3367
Postoperative pain			
(NRS max 0–10)			
Extubation	2 (0–4.5)	3 (0–6)	0.07
0–6 h	0 (0–3)	2 (0–4)	0.46
6–12 h	0 (0–2)	0 (0–2)	0.57
12–24 h	1 (0–2)	2 (0–3)	0.69
Postoperative opiates consumption			
Yes	19 (30%)	18 (29%)	0.8
No	44 (70%)	45 (71%)	
Time to first opioid (min)	30 (10–45)	30 (11–60)	0.6
Morphine consumption 0–24 h (mg)	0 (0–2)	0 (0–2)	>0.9

Values are expressed in mean ± standard deviation; median (interquartile range); number of patients (%); NRS (numeric rating scale).

Mean extubation time from admission in ICU was 191 ± 48 min in the Parasternal group and 305 ± 62 min in the Control group (Table 1).

Respiratory performance was evaluated by the TriFlo Inspiratory Exerciser and was expressed in the number of balls moved up during inspiration one hour after extubation. The median number of balls moved up was 2 (1–2) in the Parasternal group versus 1 (1–2) in the Control group.

Side effects, such as nausea, vomiting and delirium, were present in a small percentage of patients (2–3%) in both groups. Data regarding respiratory performance and side effects are reassumed in Table 3.

Table 3. Secondary Outcomes.

	Parasternal	Control	*p*-Value
Time to extubation (min)	191 ± 48	305 ± 62	**<0.001**
Pulmonary performance (balls moved up)			
Basal	3 (2–3)	3 (2–3)	0.9
After extubation	2 (1–2)	1 (1–2)	**0.045**
Side effects			
Nausea	2 (3%)	1 (2%)	–
Vomit	1 (2%)	2 (3%)	–
Delirium	1 (2%)	2 (3%)	–

Values are expressed in mean ± standard deviation; median (interquartile range); number of patients (%).

4. Discussion

This study was conducted on an extremely heterogeneous population, including every patient who underwent cardiac surgery; we tried to confront two different groups with different analgesic strategies in terms of pain management, recovery capacity and postoperative outcome.

Due to the increased life expectancy, heart surgery has become frequent in the elderly population; in our study, while the mean age of our patients was 70 years old, we faced many patients aged 80 years or more and were affected by many comorbidities. To best manage this frail population, it is mandatory to devise an anaesthetic plan aimed at minimizing the impact on the patient's vital functions and homeostasis [17]. Perioperative strategies must be adopted to reduce surgical invasiveness, post-operative pain, anaesthetic drugs usage and promote early respiratory recovery and patient-autonomous mobilization [1].

Pain, in fact, plays a central role in this therapeutic process; it reduces thoracic excursion and influences respiratory functional recovery, finally promoting pulmonary complications, such as pneumoniae, pleural effusion and lung atelectasis.

Different regional anaesthetic protocols have been proposed to better control sternal pain after cardiac surgery. Starting from neuraxial techniques, different approaches have been developed to target the thoracic fascial plane where intercostal nerves from T1 to T11 lay, such as the pectoral blocks [18,19], the serratus anterior plane block [20], the transversus thoracic muscle block [21], the erector spinae block [22] and the parasternal block. All these blocks contribute to obtaining a better control of thoracic pain in heart surgery, reducing recovery time and improving dismission time [23].

The parasternal block is one of the more promising fascial blocks to manage sternal pain as described in the recent studies conducted by Sepolvere et al. [24,25].

In our study, post-operative pain, expressed with an NRS scale from 0 to 10, was very low in both groups in absence of a significant statistical difference (Figure 2). These results are similar to the study by Lee et al. [11], as they found a marginal decrease in postoperative pain levels, although they use a longer acting local anaesthetic (liposomal bupivacaine).

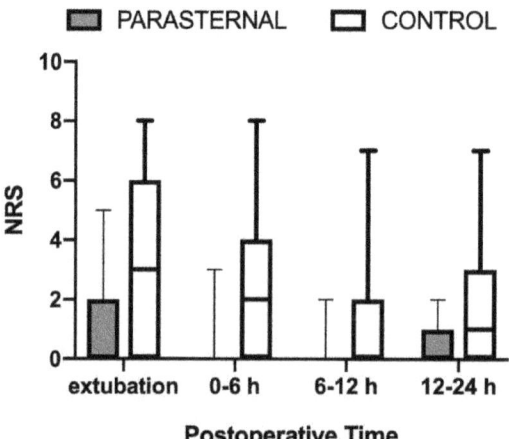

Figure 2. Postoperative Pain. *Legend:* Maximum postoperative (numeric rating scale) pain scores in both study groups reported during four postoperative intervals. Values are median (horizontal bars), IQR (box) and range (whiskers). Denotes statistical significance ($p < 0.05$).

Additionally, postoperative opiate consumption was low in both groups without any significant statistical difference, with a mean morphine consumption of 1 mg overall. This result could be correlated to the long and complex type of surgery and the timing of the block execution. In fact, we observed a mean surgical time between 3 and 4 h; moreover, a phase of recovery from anaesthesia and weaning from mechanical ventilation in ICU before weaking up was always needed. Therefore, extubation often happened several hours after the critical phase of acute postoperative pain, which is particularly intense in the immediate period after the end of the surgery, as shown in the study of Zubrzycki et al. [2]. Moreover, considering the timing of the block execution, patients were often extubated several hours after the execution of the parasternal block when the analgesic effect is not at the apex anymore, which is in accordance with the studies demonstrating that the analgesic effect of the block usually last between 5 and 12 h [26,27]. Nevertheless, the small difference in pain detected at patients awakening could have had a role in the prolonged extubation time observed in the Control group. Performing the block during the postoperatively probably impacted more on pain, but some difficulties may rise, such as the oedema of the nearby tissues and the sterile medication applied on the wound itself, which both may be complicating factors for ultrasound visualization. Moreover, and most important, performing the block before the surgery has an important impact on diminishing intraoperative opiates consumption, as demonstrated by Bloc et al. [28].

Another interesting result regards intraoperative fentanyl consumption: intraoperative administration in the Control group was twice the dose used in the Parasternal group. This result is in line with a recent study conducted in 2020 [16], which compared two groups of cardiac surgery patients who underwent parasternal block before and after the intervention. Authors found a significant reduction in intraoperative opioid administration in the preoperative Parasternal group, suggesting an important pre-emptive and intra-operative effect of the block. Limiting the intraoperative dosage of opiates could lead to rapid weaning from mechanical ventilation, early extubation and lucid weaking up, which improves patient outcomes.

Moreover, considering the low NRS scores and the successful postoperative pain control in both groups, the analgesic intraoperative regimen adopted probably had an important influence on the postoperative period. Multimodal pre-emptive analgesia with opiates, FANS, regional anaesthesia, corticosteroids, and paracetamol plays a fundamental role in preventing the development of surgical pain [29].

Notably, time to extubation could be affected by several other factors, such as preoperative conditions, i.e., pre-existing pulmonary and neurologic disorders; surgical factors, such as intraoperative and postoperative bleeding; and postoperative conditions, such as arrhythmia or bleeding. Nevertheless, we did not register significant differences in patients' characteristics and perioperative conditions that could have affected or delayed time to extubation.

It must be said that other parameters, such as intraoperative heart rate and pressure values, use of vasopressor drugs, conscious state at awakening and respiratory complications, have not been evaluated in our study.

Pulmonary performance is another interesting result to underline. Postoperative chest pain is usually evaluated with the patient in a supine position in the absence of movement. Respiratory evaluation could be a way to evaluate parasternal block efficacy when the thorax is moving.

Every patient underwent the TriFlo Inspiratory Exerciser test immediately after extubation and weaning from mechanical ventilation, which was compared to the baseline test performed immediately before surgery. Data showed that patients in the parasternal block moved up a mean of one ball more than the Control group (2 and 1 balls, respectively). This result may suggest a better analgesic effect of the parasternal block during thoracic excursions and consequently a better respiratory performance in the postoperative period; this implies better blood oxygenation and oxygen saturation, better airway clearance and a lower risk of postoperative pneumonia. Moreover, earlier extubation and less mechanical ventilation time could also have improved respiratory performance in the Parasternal group.

This study has several limitations. Firstly, it is difficult to show a clinically meaningful result for postoperative pain, which was one of our primary outcomes, when baseline postoperative pain scores are already low. However, these results confirm those of Lee et al. [11].

Secondly, we did not record pain on movement, although performance at spirometer may be considered an inversely proportional indirect index of chest pain.

Moreover, we did not investigate the correlation between perioperative analgesia and other outcomes, such as, days of ICU stay, total hospitalization time and incidence of chronic postoperative pain. At the same time, we did not correlate time to extubation and postoperative spirometer performance with the incidence of respiratory complications, leading, for example, to supplemental oxygen therapy or mechanical ventilation. We expect several future studies focus in depth on these aspects.

Another limit of the study is broad inclusion and exclusion criteria without reporting more baseline characteristics that could have influenced the primary outcome, such as pre-existing chronic pain and neuropathy, although the incidence of chronic opioid medications was similar among groups. Nevertheless, some important pre-existing conditions have been investigated and discussed.

Lastly, postoperative multimodal analgesia included on-demand administration of i.v. morphine, although recommendations indicate the oral route is preferable for opioid intake. However, this is not always possible as patients undergoing cardiothoracic surgery may have dysphagia and an increased aspiration risk in the first postoperative period [30].

In this regard, a solution could be represented by the administration of sublingual sufentanil through a patient-controlled analgesia (PCA) system, which has already proved to be effective and safe in thoracic surgery [31].

5. Conclusions

Ultrasound guided parasternal block seems to be an effective, safe and easy to perform technique in patients undergoing cardiac surgery under sternotomy. Although it did not significantly affect postoperative analgesia, it showed a relevant reduction in intraoperative opioid consumption and a better postoperative performance at spirometry compared to the Control group. Further studies are expected to confirm these findings and explore the medium- and long-term impact of this technique on postoperative morbidity.

Author Contributions: Conceptualization, G.N., A.D.P., D.S., F.C. and G.P.; methodology, G.P., F.C., A.D.C. and F.E.A.; software, M.C. (Massimiliano Carassiti) and F.E.A.; validation, F.E.A., M.C. (Massimiliano Carassiti), M.C. (Massimo Chello), R.C. and D.S.; formal analysis, L.S., G.P., A.M. and A.A.; investigation, A.D.P., G.N., A.A., D.S., G.G., L.M. and S.G.; resources, A.N. and M.C. (Massimo Chello); data curation, A.S., G.P., G.N., L.S., A.M.; writing—original draft preparation, G.N., A.S.; writing—review and editing, G.P., L.S.; visualization, G.G., L.M. and S.G.; supervision, F.C., D.S.; project administration, M.C. (Massimiliano Carassiti), R.C., F.E.A., L.M.; funding acquisition, not applicable. All authors have read and agreed to the published version of the manuscript.

Funding: This research received no external funding.

Institutional Review Board Statement: The study was conducted according to the guidelines of the Declaration of Helsinki and approved by the Institutional Review Board (or Ethics Committee) of Campus BioMedico di Roma (protocol number 20/20 PAR ComEt CBM).

Informed Consent Statement: Informed consent was obtained from all subjects involved in the study.

Data Availability Statement: The data presented in this study are available on request from the corresponding author due to privacy and ethical reasons.

Conflicts of Interest: The authors declare no conflict of interest.

References

1. White, P.F.; Kehlet, H.; Neal, J.M.; Schricker, T.; Carr, D.B.; Carli, F. The role of the anesthesiologist in fast-track surgery: From multimodal analgesia to perioperative medical care. *Anesth. Analg.* **2007**, *104*, 1380–1396. [CrossRef]
2. Zubrzycki, M.; Liebold, A.; Skrabal, C.; Reinelt, H.; Ziegler, M.; Perdas, E.; Zubrzycka, M. Assessment and pathophysiology of pain in cardiac surgery. *J. Pain. Res.* **2018**, *11*, 1599–1611. [CrossRef] [PubMed]
3. Engelman, D.T.; Ben Ali, W.; Williams, J.B.; Perrault, L.P.; Reddy, V.S.; Arora, R.C.; Roselli, E.E.; Khoynezhad, A.; Gerdisch, M.; Levy, J.H.; et al. Guidelines for Perioperative Care in Cardiac Surgery: Enhanced Recovery After Surgery Society Recommendations. *JAMA Surg.* **2019**, *154*, 755–766. [CrossRef] [PubMed]
4. Liu, H.; Emelife, P.I.; Prabhakar, A.; Moll, V.; Kendrick, J.B.; Parr, A.T.; Hyatali, F.; Pankaj, T.; Li, J.; Cornett, E.M.; et al. Regional anesthesia considerations for cardiac surgery. *Best Pract. Res. Clin. Anaesthesiol.* **2019**, *33*, 387–406. [CrossRef] [PubMed]
5. Costa, F.; Strumia, A.; Remore, L.M.; Pascarella, G.; Del Buono, R.; Tedesco, M.; Sepolvere, G.; Scimia, P.; Fusco, P. Breast surgery analgesia: Another perspective for PROSPECT guidelines. *Anaesthesia* **2020**, *75*, 1404–1405. [CrossRef] [PubMed]
6. Costa, F.; Strumia, A.; Pascarella, G.; Tomaselli, E.; Palminteri, M.; Antinolfi, V.; Montelione, N.; Stilo, F.; Spinelli, F.; Agrò, F.E. PECS II Block Combined with Supraclavicular Brachial Plexus Block Allows Anesthesia for Transaxillary Thoracic Outlet Syndrome Decompression Surgery. *J. Cardiothorac. Vasc. Anesth.* **2021**, *35*, 2234–2236. [CrossRef]

7. Grasso, A.; Orsaria, P.; Costa, F.; D'Avino, V.; Caredda, E.; Hazboun, A.; Carino, R.; Pascarella, G.; Altomare, M.; Buonomo, O.C.; et al. Ultrasound-guided Interfascial Plane Blocks for Non-anesthesiologists in Breast Cancer Surgery: Functional Outcomes and Benefits. *Anticancer Res.* **2020**, *40*, 2231–2238. [CrossRef]
8. Kar, P.; Ramachandran, G. Pain relief following sternotomy in conventional cardiac surgery: A review of non neuraxial regional nerve blocks. *Ann. Card. Anaesth.* **2020**, *23*, 200–208. [CrossRef]
9. McDonald, S.B.; Jacobsohn, E.; Kopacz, D.J.; Desphande, S.; Helman, J.D.; Salinas, F.; Hall, R.A. Parasternal block and local anesthetic infiltration with levobupivacaine after cardiac surgery with desflurane: The effect on postoperative pain, pulmonary function, and tracheal extubation times. *Anesth. Analg.* **2005**, *100*, 25–32. [CrossRef]
10. Barr, A.M.; Tutungi, E.; Almeida, A.A. Parasternal intercostal block with ropivacaine for pain management after cardiac surgery: A double-blind, randomized, controlled trial. *J. Cardiothorac. Vasc. Anesth.* **2007**, *21*, 547–553. [CrossRef]
11. Lee, C.Y.; Robinson, D.A.; Johnson, C.A., Jr.; Zhang, Y.; Wong, J.; Joshi, D.J.; Wu, T.T.; Knight, P.A. A Randomized Controlled Trial of Liposomal Bupivacaine Parasternal Intercostal Block for Sternotomy. *Ann. Thorac. Surg.* **2019**, *107*, 128–134. [CrossRef] [PubMed]
12. Doğan Bakı, E.; Kavrut Ozturk, N.; Ayoğlu, R.U.; Emmiler, M.; Karslı, B.; Uzel, H. Effects of Parasternal Block on Acute and Chronic Pain in Patients Undergoing Coronary Artery Surgery. *Semin. Cardiothorac. Vasc. Anesth.* **2016**, *20*, 205–212. [CrossRef] [PubMed]
13. Ozturk, N.K.; Baki, E.D.; Kavakli, A.S.; Sahin, A.S.; Ayoglu, R.U.; Karaveli, A.; Emmiler, M.; Inanoglu, K.; Karsli, B. Comparison of Transcutaneous Electrical Nerve Stimulation and Parasternal Block for Postoperative Pain Management after Cardiac Surgery. *Pain. Res. Manag.* **2016**, *2016*, 4261949. [CrossRef]
14. Schiavoni, L.; Nenna, A.; Cardetta, F.; Pascarella, G.; Costa, F.; Chello, M.; Agrò, F.E.; Mattei, A. Parasternal Intercostal Nerve Blocks in Patients Undergoing Cardiac Surgery: Evidence Update and Technical Considerations. *J. Cardiothorac. Vasc. Anesth.* **2022**, *36*, 4173–4182. [CrossRef] [PubMed]
15. Fusco, P.; Petrucci, E.; Marinangeli, F.; Scimia, P. Block failure or lack of efficacy? The "Double V" sign: A novel sonographic sign for a successful interfascial plane block. *Minerva Anestesiol.* **2019**, *85*, 917–918. [CrossRef]
16. Padala, S.; Badhe, A.S.; Parida, S.; Jha, A.K. Comparison of preincisional and postincisional parasternal intercostal block on postoperative pain in cardiac surgery. *J. Card. Surg.* **2020**, *35*, 1525–1530. [CrossRef]
17. Kehlet, H.; Dahl, J.B. Anaesthesia, surgery, and challenges in postoperative recovery. *Lancet* **2003**, *362*, 1921–1928. [CrossRef]
18. Blanco, R. The 'pecs block': A novel technique for providing analgesia after breast surgery. *Anaesthesia* **2011**, *66*, 847–848. [CrossRef]
19. Yalamuri, S.; Klinger, R.Y.; Bullock, W.M.; Glower, D.D.; Bottiger, B.A.; Gadsden, J.C. Pectoral Fascial (PECS) I and II Blocks as Rescue Analgesia in a Patient Undergoing Minimally Invasive Cardiac Surgery. *Reg. Anesth. Pain Med.* **2017**, *42*, 764–766. [CrossRef]
20. Khalil, A.E.; Abdallah, N.M.; Bashandy, G.M.; Kaddah, T.A. Ultrasound-Guided Serratus Anterior Plane Block Versus Thoracic Epidural Analgesia for Thoracotomy Pain. *J. Cardiothorac. Vasc. Anesth.* **2017**, *31*, 152–158. [CrossRef]
21. Fujii, S.; Roche, M.; Jones, P.M.; Vissa, D.; Bainbridge, D.; Zhou, J.R. Transversus thoracis muscle plane block in cardiac surgery: A pilot feasibility study. *Reg. Anesth. Pain Med.* **2019**, *44*, 556–560. [CrossRef] [PubMed]
22. Krishna, S.N.; Chauhan, S.; Bhoi, D.; Kaushal, B.; Hasija, S.; Sangdup, T.; Bisoi, A.K. Bilateral Erector Spinae Plane Block for Acute Post-Surgical Pain in Adult Cardiac Surgical Patients: A Randomized Controlled Trial. *J. Cardiothorac. Vasc. Anesth.* **2019**, *33*, 368–375. [CrossRef] [PubMed]
23. Kelava, M.; Alfirevic, A.; Bustamante, S.; Hargrave, J.; Marciniak, D. Regional Anesthesia in Cardiac Surgery: An Overview of Fascial Plane Chest Wall Blocks. *Anesth. Analg.* **2020**, *131*, 127–135. [CrossRef] [PubMed]
24. Sepolvere, G.; Fusco, P.; Tedesco, M.; Scimia, P. Bilateral ultrasound-guided parasternal block for postoperative analgesia in cardiac surgery: Could it be the safest strategy? *Reg. Anesth. Pain Med.* **2020**, *45*, 316–317. [CrossRef] [PubMed]
25. Sepolvere, G.; Tedesco, M.; Cristiano, L. Ultrasound Parasternal Block as a Novel Approach for Cardiac Sternal Surgery: Could it Be the Safest Strategy? *J. Cardiothorac. Vasc. Anesth.* **2020**, *34*, 2284–2286. [CrossRef]
26. Eldeen, H.M.S. Ultrasound guided pectoral nerve blockade versus thoracic spinal blockade for conservative breast surgery in cancer breast: A randomized controlled trial. *Egypt. J. Anaesth.* **2016**, *32*, 29–35. [CrossRef]
27. Kulhari, S.; Bharti, N.; Bala, I.; Arora, S.; Singh, G. Efficacy of pectoral nerve block versus thoracic paravertebral block for postoperative analgesia after radical mastectomy: A randomized controlled trial. *Br. J. Anaesth.* **2016**, *117*, 382–386. [CrossRef]
28. Bloc, S.; Perot, B.P.; Gibert, H.; Law Koune, J.D.; Burg, Y.; Leclerc, D.; Vuitton, A.S.; De La Jonquière, C.; Luka, M.; Waldmann, T.; et al. Efficacy of parasternal block to decrease intraoperative opioid use in coronary artery bypass surgery via sternotomy: A randomized controlled trial. *Reg. Anesth. Pain Med.* **2021**, *46*, 671–678. [CrossRef]

29. Wick, E.C.; Grant, M.C.; Wu, C.L. Postoperative Multimodal Analgesia Pain Management With Nonopioid Analgesics and Techniques: A Review. *JAMA Surg.* **2017**, *152*, 691–697. [CrossRef]
30. Plowman, E.K.; Anderson, A.; York, J.D.; DiBiase, L.; Vasilopoulos, T.; Arnaoutakis, G.; Beaver, T.; Martin, T.; Jeng, E.I. Dysphagia after cardiac surgery: Prevalence, risk factors, and associated outcomes. *J. Thorac. Cardiovasc. Surg.* **2021**, *165*, 737.e3–746.e3. [CrossRef]
31. Fabio, C.; Giuseppe, P.; Chiara, P.; Antongiulio, V.; Enrico, D.; Filippo, R.; Federica, B.; Eugenio, F.A. Sufentanil sublingual tablet system (Zalviso®) as an effective analgesic option after thoracic surgery: An observational study. *Saudi J. Anaesth.* **2019**, *13*, 222–226. [CrossRef] [PubMed]

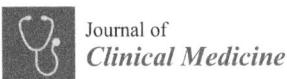

Journal of
Clinical Medicine

Article

Local Periarticular Infiltration with Dexmedetomidine Results in Superior Patient Well-Being after Total Knee Arthroplasty Compared with Peripheral Nerve Blocks: A Randomized Controlled Clinical Trial with a Follow-Up of Two Years

Patrick Reinbacher [1], Gregor A. Schittek [2], Alexander Draschl [1,3,*], Andrzej Hecker [3,4], Andreas Leithner [1], Sebastian Martin Klim [1], Kevin Brunnader [1], Amir Koutp [1], Georg Hauer [1] and Patrick Sadoghi [1]

1   Department of Orthopaedics & Traumatology, Medical University of Graz, 8036 Graz, Austria;
    patrick.reinbacher@medunigraz.at (P.R.); patrick.sadoghi@medunigraz.at (P.S.)
2   Department of Anesthesiology and Intensive Care Medicine, Medical University of Graz, 8036 Graz, Austria
3   Division of Plastic, Aesthetic and Reconstructive Surgery, Department of Surgery, Medical University of Graz,
    8036 Graz, Austria
4   COREMED—Centre for Regenerative Medicine and Precision Medicine, Joanneum Research
    Forschungsgesellschaft mbH, 8010 Graz, Austria
*   Correspondence: alexander.draschl@stud.medunigraz.at

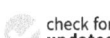

check for
updates

Citation: Reinbacher, P.; Schittek, G.A.; Draschl, A.; Hecker, A.; Leithner, A.; Klim, S.M.; Brunnader, K.; Koutp, A.; Hauer, G.; Sadoghi, P. Local Periarticular Infiltration with Dexmedetomidine Results in Superior Patient Well-Being after Total Knee Arthroplasty Compared with Peripheral Nerve Blocks: A Randomized Controlled Clinical Trial with a Follow-Up of Two Years. *J. Clin. Med.* **2023**, *12*, 5088. https://doi.org/10.3390/jcm12155088

Academic Editors: Emmanuel Andrès, Felice Eugenio Agro, Giuseppe Pascarella and Fabio Costa

Received: 26 June 2023
Revised: 27 July 2023
Accepted: 31 July 2023
Published: 2 August 2023

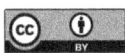
Abstract: Background: This study aimed to compare local periarticular infiltration (LIA) with ultrasound guided regional anesthesia (USRA) with ropivacaine and dexmedetomidine as an additive agent in primary total knee arthroplasty (TKA). Methods: Fifty patients were randomized into two groups in a 1:1 ratio. Patients in the LIA group received local periarticular infiltration into the knee joint. The USRA group received two single-shot USRA blocks. Functional outcomes and satisfaction (range of movement, Knee Society Knee Score, Western Ontario and McMaster Universities Osteoarthritis Index, Oxford Knee Score, and Forgotten Joint Score), including well-being, were analyzed preoperatively and at five days, six weeks, and one and two years postoperatively. Results: Functional outcomes did not significantly differ between the two groups at six weeks and one and two years after the implementation of TKA. A moderate correlation was observed in the LIA group regarding well-being and pain on day five. Six weeks postoperatively, the LIA group showed significantly superior well-being but worse pain scores. No differences between the groups in well-being and functional outcomes could be observed one and two years postoperatively. Conclusion: Patients treated with LIA had superior postoperative well-being in the early postoperative phase of up to six weeks. Furthermore, LIA patients had similar functionality compared to patients treated with USRA but experienced significantly more pain six weeks postoperatively. LIA leads to improved short-term well-being, which is potentially beneficial for faster knee recovery. We believe that LIA benefits fast-track knee recovery with respect to improved short-term well-being, higher practicability, and faster application.

Keywords: pain management; total knee arthroplasty; well-being; dexmedetomidine; local infiltration analgesia; peripheral nerve block

1. Introduction

Postoperative pain management is still developing [1] but is crucial for successful patient recovery, rehabilitation [2,3], satisfaction, and perioperative well-being [4–9]. Currently, no ideal analgesic protocol for total knee arthroplasty (TKA) performs best in all outcome measures, including well-being [10,11].

The optimization of analgesia in TKA patients plays an important role in postoperative clinical outcomes, as there is a strong association between postoperative pain, early recovery, and functionality [12]. Postoperative pain can impair recovery and hinder early rehabilitation [2,13]. As rehabilitation should start immediately after surgery, pain management in TKA should permit adequate knee movement with minimal pain and no motor blocking to accelerate early mobilization for better postoperative functionality of the affected knee [14].

In recent years, there has been a shift toward using multimodal analgesic regimens to aim at multiple pain pathways while reducing opioid consumption. Among these, multimodal pain regimens utilizing local infiltration analgesia (LIA), also known as the local periarticular infiltration anesthesia technique, and peripheral nerve blocks (PNB) have emerged to handle surgical pain and enable early postoperative mobilization [15–17].

Among peripheral nerve blocks (PNBs), the femoral, sciatic, and obturator nerves are the most common targets for postoperative analgesia by ultrasound-guided regional anesthesia (USRA) in TKA [18]. Furthermore, the combination of a femoral (FNB) and sciatic nerve block (SNB), which contributes to additional improved pain relief compared to FNB alone [19,20], is described by a recent meta-analysis as one of the best options when it comes to early pain relief [21].

However, although the combination of FNB and SNB shows excellent results in pain reduction, it is associated with reduced mobility from muscle weakness, which can prevent a rapid recovery from occurring [10,22]. This is one of the reasons that LIA has been the subject of increasing interest in recent years [23]. Besides its advantages regarding lower complication rates and reduced systemic toxicity, the application of LIA in TKA is simple and fast [15,18,24]. Moreover, the analgesic effect of both approaches is reported to be comparable, with no significant difference in the short-term, making LIA a feasible alternative to combined femoral and sciatic nerve blocks [25].

The use of perineural dexmedetomidine in combination with nerve blocks has emerged as a potentially promising approach to enhance the outcomes of regional anesthesia [26–28]. Several studies have reported positive results, including a prolonged block duration, effective postoperative pain relief, and increased patient satisfaction [26–28]. As a result, dexmedetomidine as an adjuvant has garnered attention for its potential to improve the overall patient experience during and after surgical procedures in different settings, including regional and epidural anesthesia and analgesia [29,30]. In the context of epidural analgesia and anesthesia, dexmedetomidine as an adjuvant has been subjected to a meta-analysis, confirming its general safety and tolerability. The findings suggest that dexmedetomidine can be used as a valuable adjuvant in epidural analgesia and anesthesia, providing additional benefits in terms of pain control and patient comfort [30].

Concerning regional anesthesia and analgesia, it has shown superiority over fentanyl in elective cesarean sections by increasing the time to first rescue analgesia and prolonging the duration of the sensory block [29]. Additionally, a study by Schittek et al. provided data on TKA patients who received USRA with FNB and SNB as well as LIA with dexmedetomidine as an adjuvant in both groups [18]. The authors observed significantly more pain in the USRA group than in the LIA group at rest and exercise one day after surgery, with no meaningful difference between the study groups until the sixth postoperative day [18]. Furthermore, they detected a longer-lasting opioid-sparing effect in both groups, which they attributed to the addition of dexmedetomidine.

Given these promising outcomes, dexmedetomidine has also been described as one of the most promising additive drugs in the field of regional anesthesia [31]. However, there is a lack of data regarding the impact on well-being and early functional outcomes when adding dexmedetomidine to the USRA approach with FNB and SNB or the LIA approach for TKA patients.

As LIA is a feasible alternative to USRA due to its ease of implementation and rapid placement in clinical practice, we examined these two concepts in TKA as part of this prospective randomized controlled study with a two-year follow-up. We focused on ambulation, postoperative well-being, and functional outcome scores after surgery.

This study aimed to compare local periarticular infiltration (LIA) with ultrasound-guided regional anesthesia (USRA) with ropivacaine and dexmedetomidine as an additive agent in primary total knee arthroplasty (TKA).

2. Materials and Methods

This randomized, controlled clinical trial (RCT) followed accepted ethical, scientific, and medical standards and was conducted in compliance with recognized international standards, including the principles of the Declaration of Helsinki. Informed consent was obtained from all the participants, and the study protocol was approved by the institutional Ethics Committee (32–239 ex 19/20) and registered with data safety authorities (study registry: ClinicalTrials.gov, NCT04697537).

2.1. Study Population

The study's cohort was based on a previous study [18] that examined two novel analgesic regimens for TKA using dexmedetomidine additionally in LIA and USRA, focusing on opioid consumption, postoperative pain, and complications, but was terminated due to ethical considerations. With a minimum follow-up of two years in this study population, we aimed to gain new insights into the effects of the described analgesic regimens on patients' clinical outcomes and well-being up to two years postoperatively. We included consecutive patients from February to April 2021. Adult patients with end-state osteoarthritis were included in the study. Every patient enrolled in the randomized, controlled clinical trial analysis study received an Attune TKA (DePuy Synthes, Warsaw, IN, USA) operated by the same senior surgeon. The Attune Knee system is a versatile implant system for TKA [32]. It was developed by DePuy Synthes was introduced to address concerns about anterior knee problems and high dissatisfaction rates (up to 21%) associated with the previous PFC Sigma TKA by DePuy Orthopaedics [33]. The system had a limited launch in 2011 and was formally launched in 2013 [32,34]. The new design features a femoral component with a gradually reduced radius, enhancing conformity with the polyethylene insert to allow gradual femoral rollback and greater mid-flexion stability; in addition, the marketing emphasizes the unique patellar system for improved tracking and bone coverage [35,36]. Moreover, the tibial base component integrates a central locking system, aiming to provide more secure fixation and reduce micromotion at the backside of the implant [37].

Patients were randomly assigned to the USRA or LIA group in a 1:1 ratio. A web-based randomization tool from the Institute for Medical Informatics, Statistics, and Documentation (https://www.randomizer.at, accessed on 27 November 2020, certified according to ISO-9001:2015) generated the random allocation sequence before the surgery. Patients and physicians were aware of the group assignments. In the LIA group, patients were given local infiltration analgesia from the surgeon at the end of TKA. In the USRA group, patients received two ultrasound-guided peripheral nerve blocks from their anesthesiologist immediately before anesthesia induction in the operating theater. Postoperatively, the patients followed a standardized rehabilitation protocol, which consisted of full weight bearing with crutches immediately after surgery and continuous passive motion (CPM) on the first postoperative day. The study adhered to the applicable CONSORT guidelines [38].

2.2. Local Infiltration Anesthesia Procedures and Regional Anesthesia

Patients in the LIA group received periarticular infiltration with 60 mL ropivacaine 0.5% and 1 mL dexmedetomidine (100 µg mL^{-1}) around the knee joint, including the posterior capsule, to block distal nerve fibers. The volume LIA was distributed according to the surgeon's choice. The infiltration was performed before positioning the liner and after the femoral and tibial components' implantation. Before skin closure and the end of surgery, the infiltration procedure treated the knee joint capsule, posterior joint structures, periarticular soft tissue, and subcutaneous soft tissues.

According to the local standard operating procedure, both single-shot peripheral nerve blocks were conducted in the USRA group immediately before the induction of general anesthesia or spinal anesthesia. A 120-mm 22-gauge needle (Pajunk SonoplexStim; GmbH Medizintechnologie, Geistigen, Germany) was used under sterile conditions to perform the blocks. A linear ultrasound transducer (frequency 10 to 12 MHz) was used to visualize the target nerves, the needle, and the surrounding structures.

Approximately 1–3 cm before the sciatic nerve's division into the common perineal and tibial nerves and at a safe distance from the popliteal fossa, the distal single-shot sciatic nerve was performed. The nerve block was performed in the supine position, with the foot resting on an elevated footrest. An ultrasound-guided in-line needle insertion technique was used for needle placement and control of local anesthetic spread. Perineurally, a mixture of 15 mL ropivacaine 0.5% and 0.5 mL dexmedetomidine (100 μg mL^{-1}) was injected. To reduce patient discomfort during regional anesthesia, ultrasound-guided femoral nerve blockade with the simultaneous intravenous administration of remifentanil 20 was performed before anesthetic induction. Thus, patients were placed in the supine position to access the groin. Another mixture of 15 mL ropivacaine 0.5% and 0.5 mL dexmedetomidine (100 μg mL^{-1}) was injected perineurally with an ultrasound-guided in-line needle insertion technique for proper needle placement. One senior anesthesiologist performed USRA.

2.3. Surgical Technique and Anesthetic Management

All TKA procedures were carried out by one senior knee surgeon using the same surgical technique via the medial parapatellar approach with no patella resurfacing, with an extension gap first flexion gap balanced system (Attune, DePuy Synthes, West Chesrer, PA, USA). Both the femoral and tibial components were cemented (Palacos R + G, Heraeus Medical, Wehrheim, Germany). Attending anesthesiologists were not limited in their clinical management of the patients, except that no peripheral nerve blocks were allowed in the LIA group.

2.4. Outcome Measurement

The endpoints for analysis were functional outcome parameters. The following questionnaires were used: Knee Society Knee Score (KSKS) and Knee Society Function Score (KSFS) [39], Western Ontario and McMaster Universities Osteoarthritis Index (WOMAC) [40], Oxford Knee Score (OKS) [41], Forgotten Joint Score (FJS) [42], and the English version of the "Evaluation du Vécu de l'Anesthésie LocoRégionale" (EVAN-LR) [43]. In addition, the Anästhesiolgischer Nachbefragungsbogen (ANP) [44] has been validated to assess postoperative disturbances and satisfaction. The ANP was used to determine well-being. The range of motion (ROM) was measured with a double-armed goniometer. Patients were evaluated preoperatively and 5 days, 6 weeks, 12 months, and 24 months postoperatively.

2.5. Statistical Analysis

Data were reported as numbers of patients in percent, means ($\pm$SD) for parametric data or medians (25 to 75 percentiles [IQR]) for nonparametric data, and the Kolmogorov–Smirnov and Shapiro–Wilk tests were used for normal distribution testing. For univariate analyses of statistical significance, Fisher's exact test or the Mann–Whitney test for nonparametric data were performed. Statistical significance was analyzed with a two-sided alpha of less than 5% as a significance level. Further analyses included rank correlation with Spearman's ρ and logistic regression. Spearman correlations were performed to assess a possible correlation between the use of LIA and the items of the questionnaires (at rest and during exercise). For the logistic regression models for well-being, the covariates "type of anesthesia" (general anesthesia [binary]), "type of administration of local anesthetics "(LIA [binary]), and "sex" (binary) were adjusted. The well-being Likert scores with a threshold of good (two lowest disturbance scores) and bad (two highest scores) were dichotomized in this logistic regression analysis. A priori power analysis (Statistical Solutions Ltd. nQuery Advisor Version 8.4.1 2019; Cork, Ireland) regarding the endpoints well-being and clinical outcome was performed with a difference of 10% set for clinical relevance and revealed a number of n = 25 per group as sufficient, with a *p*-value < 0.05 and a power greater than 80%. Statistical significance was analyzed with a two-sided alpha of less than 5% as a significance level. Correlations were defined as weak when r = 0.10–0.29, moderate when r = 0.30–0.59, and strong when r > 0.59 (and vice versa for negative correlations).

3. Results

Of 56 consecutive patients screened for eligibility (Figure 1), 50 were randomized and included in the final analysis. No dropouts and no complications associated with USRA or LIA were observed in this study. The characteristics of the patients did not differ but for the more frequently applied general anesthesia in the USRA group. Spinal anesthesia was more frequent in the LIA group (*p* = 0.037). No significant differences were observed between the two groups in baseline characteristics and demographics (Table 1).

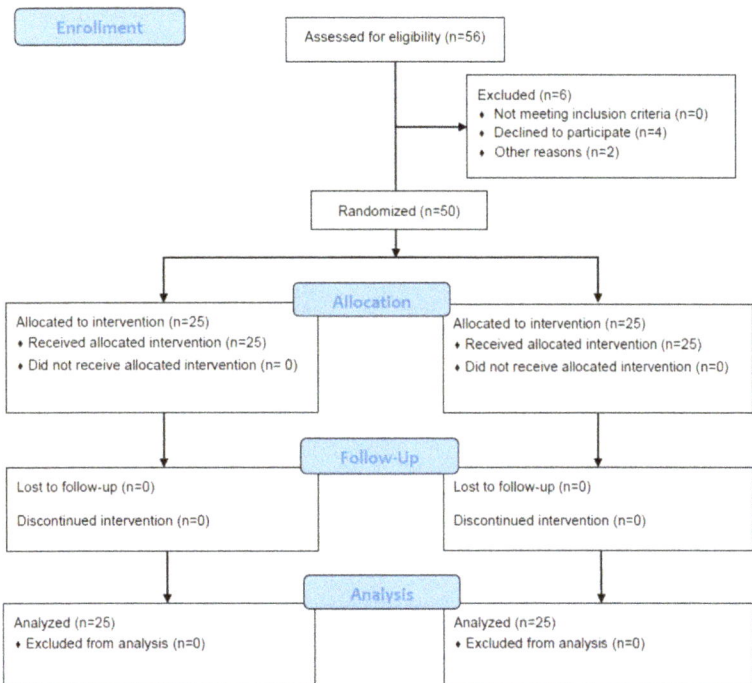

Figure 1. Study enrollment. Fifty-six consecutive patients were screened for eligibility. These patients were randomized into two groups. One group was given local periarticular infiltration anesthesia (LIA) into the knee capsule during surgery and the other was given two single-shot ultrasound-guided regional anesthesia (USRA) blocks.

3.1. Well-Being

The analysis of the questionnaires revealed that ten patients in the LIA group reported well-being, while only three did so in the USRA group, six weeks postoperatively (*p* = 0.024) (Table 1). No significant differences were found in well-being during the follow-up (*p* = 1.000).

Table 1. Patient characteristics, anesthesia, days of hospitalization, and well-being.

	USRA, N = 25	LIA, N = 25	*p*-Value
Age (years)	67.6 (±11.0)	68.6 (±10.2)	0.771
Female (%)	10 (40)	12 (48)	0.569
BMI (kg/m^2)	27.8 [24.3 to 33.8]	28.4 [25.7 to 31.6]	0.734
ASA 1 (%)	1 (4)	0 (0)	
ASA 2 (%)	7 (28)	10 (40)	0.437
ASA 3 (%)	17 (68)	15 (60)	
General anesthesia (%)	11 (44)	5 (20)	0.037
Spinal anesthesia (%)	14 (56)	20 (80)	
Days of hospitalization	6.0 [6.0 to 7.0]	6.0 [6.0 to 7.0]	0.639
Well-being, N (%)			
• Six weeks after surgery	No: 22 (88%) Yes: 3 (12%)	No: 15 (60%) Yes: 10 (40%)	0.024
• 12 months after surgery	No: 5 (11%) Yes: 42 (89%)	No: 4 (9%) Yes: 43 (91%)	1.000
• 24 months after surgery	No: 5 (11%) Yes: 42 (89%)	No: 4 (9%) Yes: 43 (91%)	1.000

LIA: local periarticular infiltration anesthesia technique; USRA: ultrasound-guided regional anesthesia; ASA: physical status classification system by the American Society of Anesthesiologists.

3.2. Functional Outcome

Functional outcome scores differed only in KSKS pain on day 5, with higher pain scores in the LIA group (*p* = 0.011). Differences in KSKS pain were non-significant thereafter. Furthermore, there were no significant differences in the other clinical outcome scores after TKA with dexmedetomidine LIA or combined FNB and SNB in the short (day 5 and week 6) or long term (one and two years), as reported in Table 2.

Table 2. Functional outcomes preoperatively and five days, six weeks, 12 months, and 24 months after primary TKA with dexmedetomidine LIA or USRA.

	USRA (n = 25)	LIA (n = 25)	*p*-Value
Range of Motion			
• Preoperative	105 [100–115]	95 [85–115]	0.412
• Five days postoperative	90 [90–100]	90 [90–100]	0.593
• Six weeks after surgery	115 [110–120]	115 [110–120]	0.734
• 12 months after surgery	118 [90–145]	119 [100–145]	0.825
• 24 months after surgery	123 [100–150]	123 [100–150]	0.241
KSKS Pain			
• Preoperative	59 [55–64]	55 [53–67]	0.464
• Five days postoperative	65 [62–67]	75 [68–92]	0.011
• Six weeks after surgery	92 [89–97]	90 [73–96]	0.907
• 12 months after surgery	96 [80–100]	95 [87–100]	0.497
• 24 months after surgery	98 [90–100]	98 [94–100]	0.189
KSKS Function			
• Preoperative	50 [50–70]	50 [50–60]	0.565
• Five days postoperative	20 [20–50]	30 [30–60]	0.257
• Six weeks after surgery	50 [50–70]	50 [50–60]	0.757
• 12 months after surgery	83 [65–100]	84 [50–100]	0.659
• 24 months after surgery	93 [65–100]	93 [80–100]	0.643

Table 2. *Cont.*

	USRA (n = 25)	LIA (n = 25)	*p*-Value
WOMAC			
• Preoperative	57.1 [54.2–63.4]	58.6 [55–62.3]	0.846
• Five days postoperative	72.3 [65.9–78]	77.4 [75.1–80.3]	0.081
• Six weeks after surgery	90.1 [85.3–94.1]	90.5 [90.3–95.3]	0.294
• 12 months after surgery	92.6 [86–100]	93.4 [86–100]	0.711
• 24 months after surgery	94.1 [90–100]	95.8 [90–100]	0.754
OKS			
• Preoperative	19 [17–23]	16 [14–22]	0.255
• Six weeks after surgery	31 [27–36]	31 [27–36]	0.712
• 12 months after surgery	38 [28–42]	37 [28–41]	0.862
• 24 months after surgery	43 [31–45]	43 [32–46]	0.897
FJS			
• Six weeks after surgery	48 [47–51]	51 [49–53]	0.090
• 12 months after surgery	62 [48–75]	63 [49–78]	0.382
• 24 months after surgery	80 [60–92]	82 [58–94]	0.827

LIA: local infiltration anesthesia; USRA: ultrasound-guided regional anesthesia (combined femoral and sciatic nerve block); ROM: range of motion; KSKS: Knee Society Knee Score; WOMAC: Western Ontario and McMaster Universities Osteoarthritis Index; OKS: Oxford Knee Score; FJS: Forgotten Joint Score.

3.3. Postoperative Improvement

Functional outcome scores differed only in KSKS pain on day 5, with higher pain scores in the LIA group (*p* = 0.011). Differences in KSKS pain were non-significant thereafter. Furthermore, there were no significant differences in the other clinical outcome scores after TKA with dexmedetomidine LIA or combined FNB and SNB in the short- (day 5 and week 6), long-term (one and two years), which is reported in Table 2.

3.4. Rank Correlation and Logistic Regression Analyses

Regarding the observed correlations between LIA and the questionnaires, only well-being and KSKS pain five days after surgery (r = 0.401, r = 0.362, *p* < 0.01) were correlated moderately. When the well-being of patients was placed in a logistic regression model adjusted for LIA, sex, and type of anesthesia (spinal or general anesthesia), only the performance of LIA remained significant (Table 3). The comparison between the USRA and LIA groups regarding return to sex (*p* = 0.231), allodynia (*p* = 0.191), and hyperalgesia (*p* = 0.280) six weeks and one and two years after surgery showed no significant differences between groups.

Table 3. Patient well-being in a logistic regression model adjusted for LIA, sex, and type of anesthesia.

	Exp (B)	95% CI for Exp (B)		*p*-Value
		Lower	Upper	
male sex	0.622	9 (50%)	30 (86%)	0.009
LIA	5.254	13 (72%)	27 (77%)	0.743
GA	0.748	4 (22%)	11 (31%)	0.539

Variables entered at step 1: male sex, local infiltration anesthesia (LIA), general anesthesia (GA). Exp (B): regression coefficient; CI: confidence interval.

4. Discussion

This study aimed to compare local periarticular infiltration (LIA) with ultrasound-guided regional anesthesia (USRA) with ropivacaine and dexmedetomidine as an additive agent in primary total knee arthroplasty (TKA).

The most important finding of our investigation was that patients reported significantly higher rates of well-being when LIA was performed than USRA, despite higher postoperative opioid requirements during the first 24 postoperative hours [18]. Although a higher rate of well-being was observed in the LIA group six weeks postoperatively, there were no differences between the two groups one and two years after TKA. Moreover, no differences in the long term could be observed concerning clinical outcomes, including pain.

This could mean that the sensory/motor block caused by USRA has a greater influence on early well-being than more intense pain and a greater need for opioids, as observed in our LIA group. We interpret this in light of the patients' expectations, which certainly include postoperative pain more often than temporary motor paralysis for up to two days postoperatively, leading to the aforementioned results. This circumstance can probably be best explained by the brief and simplified definition of well-being, ". . . the state of feeling healthy and happy", which can only be assessed subjectively [45].

It is known that general physical well-being affects satisfaction in patients following TKA [46]. Furthermore, psychological factors, such as tangible support, depression, dysfunctional coping, and low optimism, are associated with higher pain and inferior results in functionality as well as patient satisfaction after TKA [47]. Hence, we interpret this as growing evidence that well-being, including physical and mental components, appears to play a more important role than previously thought.

Kampitak et al. [48] assessed patient satisfaction in their study, in which LIA and an adductor canal block (ACB) were compared. Contradictory to our observed well-being scores, the patient satisfaction score of the LIA group was inferior to that of the USRA group; however, the difference was statistically non-significant. Kastelik et al. [49] presented comparable results in patient satisfaction and requirements for postoperative oral morphine equivalents during the hospital stay between LIA and single-shot SNB combined with ACB, which is different from our findings. Moreover, Uesugi et al. [50], comparing combined FNB and SNB with LIA, found no significant difference in satisfaction with analgesia up to 48 h after TKA. However, in the present RCT, we showed superior short-term well-being rates for LIA compared to USRA for the first time, although the LIA group experienced significantly more pain on day 5 after TKA. We see the greater well-being observed six weeks postoperatively as a psychological advantage with a potentially higher grade of motivation for rehabilitation, which could lead to improved knee recovery and overall satisfaction. Improvements in functional outcomes due to early mobilization [51–53] and the beneficial effects of LIA on functional recovery and pain control have been repeatedly described [54–57].

Regarding postoperative short-term functionality, our findings align with previous studies that evaluated patients who underwent TKA with regional anesthesia or LIA, showing no significant differences up to one year after surgery [13,58]. Fan et al. evaluated the KSKS function score up to one year after TKA in patients receiving either regional anesthesia with FNB or LIA [58]. In accordance with their results, we did not observe significant differences in short-term functionality up to one year post-TKA. Furthermore, the lack of statistically significant differences regarding postoperative short-term functionality observed in our study is consistent with the findings of Li et al. [13], who assessed patients undergoing TKA with regional anesthesia involving a combined ACB and lateral cutaneous femoral nerve block (LCFNB) versus LIA. Similar to our findings, they also did not observe a significant difference in the KSKS function score between the two groups at three months post-surgery, which is comparable with our findings six weeks to six months after surgery [13]. Hence, these results suggest that both regional anesthesia and LIA appear to be comparably effective in facilitating short-term functional recovery for patients following TKA. However, it is important to mention that, when comparing FNB with LIA, Yu et al. [57] observed significantly more falls in the FNB group during the hospital stay, potentially leading to anxiety and further hindering the early rehabilitation process [59,60].

A recent study compared the additional implementation of dexmedetomidine with ropivacaine in LIA and USRA (femoral nerve block and popliteal nerve block) and revealed a superior opioid-sparing effect in both groups, with USRA being superior to LIA when compared directly [18]. As with these findings, another study demonstrated that LIA provided better results in pain control in the early postoperative period than ACB after TKA, which was beneficial to early postoperative rehabilitation and added to patient satisfaction [56]. Aso et al. [61] described that performing LIA in addition to an FNB is an effective method for postoperative pain management after TKA. Lychagin et al. [24] compared LIA with combined FNB and SNB in TKA patients and found that the PNB only provided significantly better pain relief 4 h postoperatively, with no further significant differences in pain until the fifth day after surgery. The non-significant difference between both groups differed from our results, which showed significantly more pain on the fifth day after surgery in the LIA group.

For patient satisfaction, FNB combined with LIA was determined as the best option [38]. Studies comparing LIA (using liposomal bupivacaine (LB)) with FNB found that LIA resulted in a greater number of patients ambulating on the day of surgery and faster and better recovery of function, but similar pain relief in both groups [54,57,62,63]. Furthermore, Surdam et al. [62] showed a reduction in the LIA group's average length of hospital stay (LOS). According to Spangehl et al. [64], LIA provides comparable pain relief to single-shot SNB combined with an indwelling femoral nerve catheter and results in a slightly reduced length of hospital stay.

The results of LIA and various types of USRA in terms of functional outcomes, postoperative pain, length of hospital stay, satisfaction, and opioid consumption are still controversial in the current literature [48,55–57,62,65], and it seems rather impossible to point out an intervention that performs the best in all outcome measures. Furthermore, the lack of consistency in functional outcomes may be attributable to the heterogeneity of the used agents and perioperative pain management, as well as differences in the implemented interventions in previous studies. This makes it challenging to determine whether LIA or USRA is superior for TKA in clinical practice regarding functional outcomes, early postoperative pain, and well-being.

This RCT observed that USRA and LIA influence patient well-being and early postoperative pain differently but show similar functional outcomes. We emphasize that the decision regarding whether to perform LIA or USRA should be sought individually, primarily depending on the medical indications, patient expectations, and perceptions, including the careful evaluation of individual risk factors and benefits for each patient, as well as the goals of the rehabilitation process after surgery. Our results suggest that determining the postoperative analgesic method of choice in TKA patients should also rely on whether analgesia (USRA) or motor function (LIA) is the priority, especially in the early postoperative period, to improve patient outcomes.

5. Limitations

We wish to underline that the discrepancy between spinal and general anesthesia, with more LIA patients having undergone spinal anesthesia, was a confounder within the data. Moreover, this study did not compare outcomes during the first four postoperative days, which would likely have provided additional valuable information for the comparison between the two groups, as the effects of the agents used typically disappeared after the first or second postoperative day. The observed differences among both groups (LIA vs. USRA) were based on the study's small sample size, and the results should therefore be interpreted with caution. Based on the study's limitations, we cannot suggest one method over the other as both approaches have advantages and disadvantages when it comes to well-being and pain in the early postoperative period.

6. Conclusions

Patients treated with LIA had superior postoperative well-being in the early postoperative phase of up to 6 weeks and had similar functionality in comparison to patients treated with USRA but experienced significantly more pain. LIA leads to improved short-term well-being, which is potentially beneficial for faster knee recovery, including the motivation for

J. Clin. Med. **2023**, *12*, 5088

rehabilitation and physical therapy. Additionally, LIA has advantages in its practicability, as it is easier and faster to perform than USRA.

Author Contributions: Conceptualization, P.R., G.A.S. and P.S.; methodology, P.R., G.A.S. and P.S.; validation, A.L., G.H. and P.S.; formal analysis, G.A.S. and A.H.; investigation, G.A.S., A.D., S.M.K., K.B., A.K. and G.H.; resources, G.A.S., A.L. and P.S.; data curation, K.B., A.K. and G.H.; writing—original draft preparation, P.R., G.A.S. and A.D.; writing—review and editing, A.H. and S.M.K.; visualization, A.D.; supervision, P.S. and A.L.; project administration, G.A.S. and P.S.; funding acquisition, P.S. All authors have read and agreed to the published version of the manuscript.

Funding: This work was supported by the City of Graz, Cultural Office (grant number: A16-013786/2010/0043).

Institutional Review Board Statement: The study was conducted in accordance with the Declaration of Helsinki and approved by the Institutional Review Board (or Ethics Committee) of the Medical University of Graz (32-239 ex 19/20) and registered with data safety authorities (study registry: ClinicalTrials.gov, NCT04697537).

Informed Consent Statement: Patient consent was waived due to the retrospective nature of the study.

Data Availability Statement: The datasets generated and/or analyzed during the current study are available from the corresponding author upon reasonable request.

Conflicts of Interest: A.L. received institutional and educational grants from DePuy Synthes Johnson & Johnson, Alphamed, and Medacta without relation to the submitted work. The remaining authors declare that they have no competing interests.

References

1. Elmofty, D.H.; Buvanendran, A. Regional Anesthesia in Total Joint Arthroplasty: What Is the Evidence? *J. Arthroplast.* **2017**, *32*, S74–S76. [CrossRef] [PubMed]
2. Elmallah, R.K.; Cherian, J.J.; Pierce, T.P.; Jauregui, J.J.; Harwin, S.F.; Mont, M.A. New and Common Perioperative Pain Management Techniques in Total Knee Arthroplasty. *J. Knee Surg.* **2016**, *29*, 169–178. [CrossRef]
3. Baratta, J.L.; Gandhi, K.; Viscusi, E.R. Perioperative pain management for total knee arthroplasty. *J. Surg. Orthop. Adv.* **2014**, *23*, 22–36. [CrossRef] [PubMed]
4. Schittek, G.A.; Michaeli, K.; Labmayr, V.; Reinbacher, P.; Gebauer, D.; Smigaj, J.; Gollowitsch, J.; Rief, M.; Sampl, L.; Sandner-Kiesling, A.; et al. Influence of personalised music and ice-tea options on post-operative well-being in the post anaesthesia care unit after general or regional anaesthesia. A pre-post-analysis by means of a questionnaire. *Intensiv. Crit. Care Nurs.* **2021**, *63*, 102998. [CrossRef] [PubMed]
5. Schittek, G.A.; Simonis, H.; Bornemann-Cimenti, H. Pain, nausea, vomiting, thirst, cold, . . . the challenge of well-being in post-operative patients. *Intensiv. Crit. Care Nurs.* **2021**, *66*, 103090. [CrossRef] [PubMed]
6. Schittek, G.A.; Schwantzer, G.; Simonis, H.; Heschl, S.; Sandner-Kiesling, A.; Bornemann-Cimenti, H. Randomised controlled pilot trial of concepts for analgesia and sedation during placement of peripheral regional anaesthesia before operations. *Eur. J. Anaesthesiol.* **2021**, *38*, 183–184. [CrossRef]
7. Hamilton, D.F.; Lane, J.V.; Gaston, P.; Patton, J.T.; MacDonald, D.; Simpson, A.H.R.W.; Howie, C.R. What determines patient satisfaction with surgery? A prospective cohort study of 4709 patients following total joint replacement. *BMJ Open* **2013**, *3*, e002525. [CrossRef]
8. Schittek, G.A.; Schwantzer, G.; Zoidl, P.; Orlob, S.; Holger, S.; Eichinger, M.; Sampl, L.; Bornemann-Cimenti, H.; Sandner-Kiesling, A. Adult patients' wellbeing and disturbances during early recovery in the post anaesthesia care unit. A cross-sectional study. *Intensiv. Crit. Care Nurs.* **2020**, *61*, 102912. [CrossRef]
9. Shi, Z.B.; Dang, X.Q. Efficacy of multimodal perioperative analgesia protocol with periarticular medication injection and nonsteroidal anti-inflammatory drug use in total knee arthroplasty. *Niger. J. Clin. Pract.* **2018**, *21*, 1221–1227.
10. Lavand'homme, P.M.; Kehlet, H.; Rawal, N.; Joshi, G.P. Pain management after total knee arthroplasty: PROcedure SPEcific Postoperative Pain ManagemenT recommendations. *Eur. J. Anaesthesiol.* **2022**, *39*, 743–757. [CrossRef]
11. Joshi, G.P.; Kehlet, H.; PROSPECT Working Group. Guidelines for perioperative pain management: Need for re-evaluation. *Br. J. Anaesth.* **2017**, *119*, 703–706. [CrossRef] [PubMed]
12. Parvataneni, H.K.; Shah, V.P.; Howard, H.; Cole, N.; Ranawat, A.S.; Ranawat, C.S. Controlling pain after total hip and knee arthroplasty using a multimodal protocol with local periarticular injections: A prospective randomized study. *J. Arthroplast.* **2007**, *22*, 33–38. [CrossRef] [PubMed]

13. Li, D.; Alqwbani, M.; Wang, Q.; Yang, Z.; Liao, R.; Kang, P. Ultrasound-guided adductor canal block combined with lateral femoral cutaneous nerve block for post-operative analgesia following total knee arthroplasty: A prospective, double-blind, randomized controlled study. *Int. Orthop.* **2021**, *45*, 1421–1429. [CrossRef]
14. Fu, H.; Wang, J.; Zhang, W.; Cheng, T.; Zhang, X. Potential superiority of periarticular injection in analgesic effect and early mobilization ability over femoral nerve block following total knee arthroplasty. *Knee Surg. Sports Traumatol. Arthrosc.* **2017**, *25*, 291–298. [CrossRef]
15. Keijsers, R.; van Delft, R.; Bekerom, M.P.J.v.D.; de Vries, D.C.A.A.; Brohet, R.M.; Nolte, P.A. Local infiltration analgesia following total knee arthroplasty: Effect on post-operative pain and opioid consumption—A meta-analysis. *Knee Surg. Sports Traumatol. Arthrosc.* **2015**, *23*, 1956–1963. [CrossRef] [PubMed]
16. Terkawi, A.S.; Mavridis, D.; Sessler, D.I.; Nunemaker, M.S.; Doais, K.S.; Terkawi, R.S.; Terkawi, Y.S.; Petropoulou, M.; Nemergut, E.C. Pain Management Modalities after Total Knee Arthroplasty: A Network Meta-analysis of 170 Randomized Controlled Trials. *Anesthesiology* **2017**, *126*, 923–937. [CrossRef]
17. Soffin, E.M.; Memtsoudis, S.G. Anesthesia and analgesia for total knee arthroplasty. *Minerva Anestesiol.* **2018**, *84*, 1406–1412. [CrossRef] [PubMed]
18. Schittek, G.A.; Reinbacher, P.; Rief, M.; Gebauer, D.; Leithner, A.; Vielgut, I.; Labmayr, V.; Simonis, H.; Köstenberger, M.; Bornemann-Cimenti, H.; et al. Combined femoral and popliteal nerve block is superior to local periarticular infiltration anaesthesia for postoperative pain control after total knee arthroplasty. *Knee Surgery Sports Traumatol. Arthrosc.* **2022**, *30*, 4046–4053. [CrossRef]
19. Danninger, T.; Opperer, M.; Memtsoudis, S.G. Perioperative pain control after total knee arthroplasty: An evidence based review of the role of peripheral nerve blocks. *World J. Orthop.* **2014**, *5*, 225–232. [CrossRef]
20. Abdallah, F.W.; Chan, V.W.S.; Gandhi, R.; Koshkin, A.; Abbas, S.; Brull, R. The analgesic effects of proximal, distal, or no sciatic nerve block on posterior knee pain after total knee arthroplasty: A double-blind placebo-controlled randomized trial. *Anesthesiology* **2014**, *121*, 1302–1310. [CrossRef]
21. Qin, L.; You, D.; Zhao, G.; Li, L.; Zhao, S. A comparison of analgesic techniques for total knee arthroplasty: A network meta-analysis. *J. Clin. Anesthesia* **2021**, *71*, 110257. [CrossRef] [PubMed]
22. Memtsoudis, S.G.; Danninger, T.; Rasul, R.; Poeran, J.; Gerner, P.; Stundner, O.; Mariano, E.R.; Mazumdar, M. Inpatient falls after total knee arthroplasty: The role of anesthesia type and peripheral nerve blocks. *Anesthesiology* **2014**, *120*, 551–563. [CrossRef] [PubMed]
23. Li, J.; Ma, Y.; Xiao, L. Postoperative Pain Management in Total Knee Arthroplasty. *Orthop. Surg.* **2019**, *11*, 755–761. [CrossRef]
24. Lychagin, A.V.; Gritsyuk, A.A.; Rosenberg, N.; Ceo, S.M.L. Postoperative Pain Control by Local Infiltration Analgesia and Peripheral Nerve Block in Primary Prosthetic Total Knee Arthroplasty. *Rambam Maimonides Med. J.* **2022**, *13*, e0019. [CrossRef]
25. Tian, Y.; Tang, S.; Sun, S.; Zhang, Y.; Chen, L.; Xia, D.; Wang, Y.; Ren, L.; Huang, Y. Comparison between local infiltration analgesia with combined femoral and sciatic nerve block for pain management after total knee arthroplasty. *J. Orthop. Surg. Res.* **2020**, *15*, 41. [CrossRef] [PubMed]
26. Lee, J.J.; Kim, D.-Y.; Hwang, J.-T.; Song, D.-K.; Na Lee, H.; Jang, J.S.; Lee, S.-S.; Hwang, S.M.; Moon, S.H.; Shim, J.-H. Dexmedetomidine combined with suprascapular nerve block and axillary nerve block has a synergistic effect on relieving postoperative pain after arthroscopic rotator cuff repair. *Knee Surgery Sports Traumatol. Arthrosc.* **2021**, *29*, 4022–4031. [CrossRef] [PubMed]
27. Wang, C.; Zhang, Z.; Ma, W.; Liu, R.; Li, Q.; Li, Y. Perineural Dexmedetomidine Reduces the Median Effective Concentration of Ropivacaine for Adductor Canal Block. *Med. Sci. Monit.* **2021**, *27*, e929857. [CrossRef]
28. Herman, J.; Urits, I.; Eskander, J.; Kaye, A.; Viswanath, O. Adductor Canal Block Duration of Analgesia Successfully Prolonged With Perineural Dexmedetomidine and Dexamethasone in Addition to IPACK Block for Total Knee Arthroplasty. *Cureus* **2020**, *12*, e10566. [CrossRef]
29. LA Via, L.; Santonocito, C.; Bartolotta, N.; Lanzafame, B.; Morgana, A.; Continella, C.; Cirica, G.; Astuto, M.; Sanfilippo, F. α-2 agonists vs. fentanyl as adjuvants for spinal anesthesia in elective cesarean section: A meta-analysis. *Minerva Anestesiol.* **2023**, *89*, 445–454. Available online: https://www.minervamedica.it/index2.php?show=R02Y2023N05A0445 (accessed on 25 July 2023). [CrossRef]
30. Zhang, X.; Wang, D.; Shi, M.; Luo, Y. Efficacy and Safety of Dexmedetomidine as an Adjuvant in Epidural Analgesia and Anesthesia: A Systematic Review and Meta-analysis of Randomized Controlled Trials. *Clin. Drug Investig.* **2017**, *37*, 343–354. Available online: http://link.springer.com/10.1007/s40261-016-0477-9 (accessed on 25 July 2023). [CrossRef]
31. Marhofer, P.; Brummett, C.M. Safety and efficiency of dexmedetomidine as adjuvant to local anesthetics. *Curr. Opin. Anaesthesiol.* **2016**, *29*, 632–637. Available online: https://journals.lww.com/00001503-201610000-00020 (accessed on 25 July 2023). [CrossRef] [PubMed]
32. Fisher, D.A.; David, P. Advancing Patient Outcomes and Economic Value in Total Knee Arthroplasty: The Evidence of the ATTUNE®Knee System. 2020. Available online: https://www.jnjmedtech.com/system/files/pdf/164232-210110_137851-200422_ATTUNE_Evidence.pdf (accessed on 25 July 2023).
33. Meftah, M.; Ranawat, A.S.; Ranawat, C.S. Ten-Year Follow-up of a Rotating-Platform, Posterior-Stabilized Total Knee Arthroplasty. *J. Bone Jt. Surg.* **2012**, *94*, 426–432. Available online: https://journals.lww.com/00004623-201203070-00006 (accessed on 25 July 2023). [CrossRef] [PubMed]

34. Prodromidis, A.D.; Chloros, G.D.; Thivaios, G.C.; Sutton, P.M.; Pandit, H.; Giannoudis, P.V.; Charalambous, C.P. High rate of radiolucent lines following the cemented original design of the ATTUNE total knee arthroplasty. *Bone Jt. J.* **2023**, *105-B*, 610–621. Available online: https://boneandjoint.org.uk/doi/10.1302/0301-620X.105B6.BJJ-2022-0675.R1 (accessed on 25 July 2023).

35. Indelli, P.F.; Marcucci, M.; Pipino, G.; Charlton, S.; Carulli, C.; Innocenti, M. The Effects of Femoral Component Design on the Patello-Femoral Joint in a PS Total Knee Arthroplasty. *Arch. Orthop. Trauma Surg.* **2014**, *134*, 59–64. [CrossRef]

36. Clary, C.W.; Fitzpatrick, C.K.; Maletsky, L.P.; Rullkoetter, P.J. The Influence of Total Knee Arthroplasty Geometry on Mid-Flexion Stability: An Experimental and Finite Element Study. *J. Biomech.* **2013**, *46*, 1351–1357. [CrossRef] [PubMed]

37. Cerquiglini, A.; Henckel, J.; Hothi, H.; Allen, P.; Lewis, J.; Eskelinen, A.; Skinner, J.; Hirschmann, M.T.; Hart, A.J. Analysis of the Attune Tibial Tray Backside: A Comparative Retrieval Study. *Bone Jt. Res.* **2019**, *8*, 136–145. [CrossRef] [PubMed]

38. Schulz, K.F.; Altman, D.G.; Moher, D.; CONSORT Group. CONSORT 2010 Statement: Updated guidelines for reporting parallel group randomised trials. *BMC Med.* **2010**, *8*, 18. [CrossRef]

39. Insall, J.N.; Dorr, L.D.; Scott, R.D.; Scott, W.N. Rationale of the Knee Society clinical rating system. *Clin. Orthop. Relat. Res.* **1989**, *248*, 13–14. [CrossRef]

40. Bellamy, N.; Buchanan, W.W.; Goldsmith, C.H.; Campbell, J.; Stitt, L.W. Validation study of WOMAC: A health status instrument for measuring clinically important patient relevant outcomes to antirheumatic drug therapy in patients with osteoarthritis of the hip or knee. *J. Rheumatol.* **1988**, *15*, 1833–1840.

41. Xie, F.; Ye, H.; Zhang, Y.; Liu, X.; Lei, T.; Li, S.-C. Extension from inpatients to outpatients: Validity and reliability of the Oxford Knee Score in measuring health outcomes in patients with knee osteoarthritis. *Int. J. Rheum. Dis.* **2011**, *14*, 206–210. [CrossRef]

42. Thomsen, M.G.; Latifi, R.; Kallemose, T.; Barfod, K.W.; Husted, H.; Troelsen, A. Good validity and reliability of the forgotten joint score in evaluating the outcome of total knee arthroplasty. *Acta Orthop.* **2016**, *87*, 280–285. [CrossRef]

43. Maurice-Szamburski, A.; Bruder, N.; Loundou, A.; Capdevila, X.; Auquier, P. Development and validation of a perioperative satisfaction questionnaire in regional anesthesia. *Anesthesiology* **2013**, *118*, 78–87. [CrossRef] [PubMed]

44. Beckhoff, M.; Klotz, K.-F.; Heinzinger, M.; Gerlach, K.; Ocker, H.; Schmucker, P.; Hüppe, M.; Prüßmann, M. Reliability and validity of the Anaesthesiological Questionnaire for electively operated patients. *Anaesthesist* **2003**, *52*, 311–320. [CrossRef]

45. Simons, G.; Baldwin, D.S. A critical review of the definition of 'wellbeing' for doctors and their patients in a post COVID-19 era. *Int. J. Soc. Psychiatry* **2021**, *67*, 984–991. [CrossRef]

46. Clement, N.D.; Burnett, R. Patient satisfaction after total knee arthroplasty is affected by their general physical well-being. *Knee Surgery Sports Traumatol. Arthrosc.* **2013**, *21*, 2638–2646. [CrossRef]

47. Lopez-Olivo, M.A.; Ingleshwar, A.; Landon, G.C.; Siff, S.J.; Barbo, A.; Lin, H.Y.; Suarez-Almazor, M.E. Psychosocial Determinants of Total Knee Arthroplasty Outcomes Two Years After Surgery. *ACR Open Rheumatol.* **2020**, *2*, 573–581. [CrossRef] [PubMed]

48. Kampitak, W.; Tanavalee, A.; Ngarmukos, S.; Amarase, C.; Songthamwat, B.; Boonshua, A. Comparison of Adductor Canal Block Versus Local Infiltration Analgesia on Postoperative Pain and Functional Outcome after Total Knee Arthroplasty: A Randomized Controlled Trial. *Malays. Orthop. J.* **2018**, *12*, 7–14. [CrossRef]

49. Kastelik, J.; Fuchs, M.; Krämer, M.; Trauzeddel, R.F.; Ertmer, M.; von Roth, P.; Perka, C.; Kirschbaum, S.M.; Tafelski, S.; Treskatsch, S. Local infiltration anaesthesia versus sciatic nerve and adductor canal block for fast-track knee arthroplasty: A randomised controlled clinical trial. *Eur. J. Anaesthesiol.* **2019**, *36*, 255–263. [CrossRef]

50. Uesugi, K.; Kitano, N.; Kikuchi, T.; Sekiguchi, M.; Konno, S.-I. Comparison of peripheral nerve block with periarticular injection analgesia after total knee arthroplasty: A randomized, controlled study. *Knee* **2014**, *21*, 848–852. [CrossRef]

51. Hertog, A.D.; Gliesche, K.; Timm, J.; Mühlbauer, B.; Zebrowski, S. Pathway-controlled fast-track rehabilitation after total knee arthroplasty: A randomized prospective clinical study evaluating the recovery pattern, drug consumption, and length of stay. *Arch. Orthop. Trauma Surg.* **2012**, *132*, 1153–1163. [CrossRef]

52. Henderson, K.G.; Wallis, J.A.; Snowdon, D.A. Active physiotherapy interventions following total knee arthroplasty in the hospital and inpatient rehabilitation settings: A systematic review and meta-analysis. *Physiotherapy* **2018**, *104*, 25–35. [CrossRef]

53. Castorina, S.; Guglielmino, C.; Castrogiovanni, P.; Szychlinska, M.A.; Ioppolo, F.; Massimino, P.; Leonardi, P.; Maci, C.; Iannuzzi, M.; Di Giunta, A.; et al. Clinical evidence of traditional vs fast track recovery methodologies after total arthroplasty for osteoarthritic knee treatment. A retrospective observational study. *Muscles Ligaments Tendons J.* **2017**, *7*, 504–513. [CrossRef] [PubMed]

54. Lützner, J.; Gehring, R.; Beyer, F. Slightly better pain relief but more frequently motor blockade with combined nerve block analgesia compared to continuous intraarticular analgesia after total knee arthroplasty. *Knee Surgery Sports Traumatol. Arthrosc.* **2020**, *28*, 1169–1176. [CrossRef] [PubMed]

55. Perlas, A.; Kirkham, K.R.; Billing, R.; Tse, C.; Brull, R.; Gandhi, R.; Chan, V.W.S. The impact of analgesic modality on early ambulation following total knee arthroplasty. *Reg. Anesthesia Pain Med.* **2013**, *38*, 334–339. [CrossRef] [PubMed]

56. Kulkarni, M.M.; Dadheech, A.N.; Wakankar, H.M.; Ganjewar, N.V.; Hedgire, S.S.; Pandit, H.G. Randomized Prospective Comparative Study of Adductor Canal Block vs Periarticular Infiltration on Early Functional Outcome after Unilateral Total Knee Arthroplasty. *J. Arthroplast.* **2019**, *34*, 2360–2364. [CrossRef]

57. Yu, S.; Szulc, A.; Walton, S.; Bosco, J.; Iorio, R. Pain Control and Functional Milestones in Total Knee Arthroplasty: Liposomal Bupivacaine versus Femoral Nerve Block. *Clin. Orthop. Relat. Res.* **2017**, *475*, 110–117. [CrossRef]

58. Fan, L.; Yu, X.; Zan, P.; Liu, J.; Ji, T.; Li, G. Comparison of Local Infiltration Analgesia with Femoral Nerve Block for Total Knee Arthroplasty: A Prospective, Randomized Clinical Trial. *J. Arthroplast.* **2015**, *31*, 1361–1365. Available online: https://linkinghub.elsevier.com/retrieve/pii/S0883540315011092 (accessed on 25 July 2023).
59. Theunissen, M.; Peters, M.L.; Bruce, J.; Gramke, H.-F.; Marcus, M.A. Preoperative Anxiety and Catastrophizing. *Clin. J. Pain* **2012**, *28*, 819–841. Available online: https://journals.lww.com/00002508-201211000-00010 (accessed on 25 July 2023). [CrossRef]
60. Jack, K.; McLean, S.M.; Moffett, J.K.; Gardiner, E. Barriers to treatment adherence in physiotherapy outpatient clinics: A systematic review. *Man. Ther.* **2010**, *15*, 220–228. Available online: https://linkinghub.elsevier.com/retrieve/pii/S1356689X09002094 (accessed on 25 July 2023). [CrossRef]
61. Aso, K.; Izumi, M.; Sugimura, N.; Okanoue, Y.; Kamimoto, Y.; Yokoyama, M.; Ikeuchi, M. Additional benefit of local infiltration of analgesia to femoral nerve block in total knee arthroplasty: Double-blind randomized control study. *Knee Surgery Sports Traumatol. Arthrosc.* **2019**, *27*, 2368–2374. [CrossRef]
62. Surdam, J.W.; Licini, D.J.; Baynes, N.T.; Arce, B.R. The use of exparel (liposomal bupivacaine) to manage postoperative pain in unilateral total knee arthroplasty patients. *J. Arthroplast.* **2015**, *30*, 325–329. [CrossRef]
63. Essving, P.; Axelsson, K.; Kjellberg, J.; Wallgren, A.; Gupta, A.; Lundin, A. Reduced morphine consumption and pain intensity with local infiltration analgesia (LIA) following total knee arthroplasty. *Acta Orthop.* **2010**, *81*, 354–360. [CrossRef] [PubMed]
64. Spangehl, M.J.; Clarke, H.D.; Hentz, J.G.; Misra, L.; Blocher, J.L.; Seamans, D.P. The Chitranjan Ranawat Award: Periarticular injections and femoral & sciatic blocks provide similar pain relief after TKA: A randomized clinical trial. *Clin. Orthop. Relat. Res.* **2015**, *473*, 45–53. [CrossRef] [PubMed]
65. Cicekci, F.; Yildirim, A.; Önal„ Ö.; Celik, J.B.; Kara, I. Ultrasound-guided adductor canal block using levobupivacaine versus periarticular levobupivacaine infiltration after total knee arthroplasty: A randomized clinical trial. *Sao Paulo Med. J.* **2019**, *137*, 45–53. [CrossRef] [PubMed]

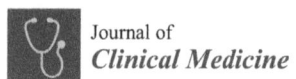

Journal of
Clinical Medicine

Article

The Effect of Cold Application to the Lateral Neck Area on Peripheral Vascular Access Pain: A Randomised Controlled Study

Senay Canikli Adıgüzel [1,*], Dilan Akyurt [1], Gökçe Ültan Özgen [1], Hatice Bahadır Altun [1], Aleyna Çakır [1], Mustafa Süren [1] and İsmail Okan [2]

[1] Samsun Training and Research Hospital, Samsun University, 55090 Samsun, Turkey; dilanakyurt@gmail.com (D.A.); gokce_ultan@yahoo.co.uk (G.Ü.Ö.); haticebahadirmd@hotmail.com (H.B.A.); aleynackr63@gmail.com (A.Ç.); mustafa.suren@samsun.edu.tr (M.S.)
[2] İstanbul Medeniyet University, 34720 Istanbul, Turkey; ismail.okan@medeniyet.edu.tr
* Correspondence: drsenaycanikli@yahoo.com

Abstract: Introduction: Various types of vagus nerve stimulation are employed in the treatment of a range of conditions, including depression, anxiety, epilepsy, headache, tinnitus, atrial fibrillation, schizophrenia, and musculoskeletal pain. The objective of this study was to apply vagal stimulation to the neck area using standardised cold, and then analyse the level of vascular access discomfort experienced by individuals who underwent venous cannulation from the dorsal side of the hand prior to anaesthesia. Materials and Methods: A total of 180 patients, aged 18–75, who were scheduled to undergo elective surgery, were categorised into three distinct groups: the Sham group (Group S), the Control group (Group K), and the Cold group (Group M), with each group consisting of 60 individuals. Bilateral cold application to the lateral side of the neck was performed prior to the commencement of vascular access in Group M patients, followed by the subsequent opening of vascular access. The alterations in heart rate among patients was assessed subsequent to the application of cold and following the establishment of vascular access. The participants were instructed to assess their level of vascular access pain on a numerical pain scale (NRS) ranging from 0 to 10. Results: A statistically significant difference ($p = 0.035$) was seen when comparing the pain ratings of patients during vascular access. The study revealed that the NRS values exhibited a statistically significant decrease in Group M compared to both Group K ($p = 0.038$) and Group S ($p = 0.048$). Group M had a higher prevalence of individuals experiencing mild pain compared to other groups, and the difference was statistically significant ($p = 0.029$). In Group M, the average heart rate following vagal stimulation exhibited a statistically significant decrease compared to the average heart rate observed at the beginning of the study ($p < 0.05$). Upon comparing the original heart rate measurements with the heart rate values following vascular access, it was observed that there was an elevation in heart rate for both Group S and Group K. Conversely, Group M exhibited a decrease in heart rate after vascular access when compared to the initial heart rate values. Conclusions: In the present investigation, it was discovered that the application of cold to the neck region resulted in a drop in heart rate among the patients, which persisted throughout the process of vascular access. Furthermore, the level of pain experienced by these individuals was reduced during vascular access procedures.

Keywords: vascular access pain; heart rate; cold application; vagal stimulation

Citation: Canikli Adıgüzel, S.; Akyurt, D.; Ültan Özgen, G.; Bahadır Altun, H.; Çakır, A.; Süren, M.; Okan, İ. The Effect of Cold Application to the Lateral Neck Area on Peripheral Vascular Access Pain: A Randomised Controlled Study. *J. Clin. Med.* 2023, 12, 6273. https://doi.org/10.3390/jcm12196273

Academic Editors: Felice Eugenio Agro, Giuseppe Pascarella, Fabio Costa and Chun Yang

Received: 28 August 2023
Revised: 21 September 2023
Accepted: 26 September 2023
Published: 28 September 2023

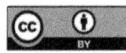
1. Introduction

The vagus nerve (N. vagus) extends from the brain stem to the proximal two-thirds of the large intestine and is therefore the longest of the cranial nerves [1]. Furthermore, apart from serving as the primary neuron of the autonomic parasympathetic system, it also has anti-inflammatory and analgesic characteristics. The afferent branch of the N. vagus can be found in the region of the ear known as the 'cymba conchae', while the cervical branch is densely situated in the neck region [2]. These regions are employed to deliver stimuli for the vagus stimulation approach. The vagus stimulation approach, formerly employed for managing refractory epilepsy, has been found to have pain-reducing effects in musculoskeletal disorders [3]. Similarly, Eastern medicine has, for millennia, harnessed the analgesic properties of auricular acupuncture [4].

The clinical application of vagus stimulation extends beyond the treatment of depression, epilepsy, and vascular access pain in encompassing additional conditions such as headache, tinnitus, atrial fibrillation, schizophrenia, and various pain management approaches. Transcutaneous cervical vagus stimulation (TCVS) is a frequently utilised non-invasive method [5]. The Valsalva manoeuvre is a physiological technique that elicits activation of the vagus nerve. It is believed that the activation of the vagal nerve by the stimulation of the baroreceptor reflex arc leads to the release of a substance similar to substance P, which exhibits antinociceptive properties [6–8]. The application of ice to the lateral neck region is believed to elicit stimulation of the vagus nerve, resulting in a reduction in heart rate. The application of cold to the neck region also leads to an antinociceptive effect, which is attributed to the activation of the parasympathetic system by the stimulation of the baroreceptor reflex arc via vagal stimulation [7].

Intravenous (IV) cannulation is a frequently employed procedure conducted by anaesthesiologists both within and beyond the confines of the operating room. Prior to the initiation of any surgery, it is imperative to establish vascular access. The process of venous cannulation is associated with a moderate level of pain, causing discomfort and heightened stress levels among patients [9]. During the venous cannulation procedure, patients' stress level and pain may increase, especially in repeated interventions. For this reason, ultrasonography support is also used to increase the success rate of cannulation and aid in single-attempt success [10,11]. Numerous methodologies have been employed in attempts to mitigate the discomfort associated with venous cannulation and to alleviate the patient's pain and divert their attention. These include the administration of local anaesthetic through injection to the intervention site, the application of topical anaesthetic, the use of cold, and the use of a vibrating buzzy device. The administration of local anaesthetic mostly alleviates the physical aspect of pain, whereas the Valsalva manoeuvre, which involves the stimulation of the vagus nerve, mitigates both the somatic and psychological dimensions of pain [8]. The induction of antinociception can be achieved through the activation of the cardiopulmonary baroreceptor reflex arc or sino-aortic baroreceptor reflex arc via the Valsalva manoeuvre. It has been noted that the elevation of intrathoracic pressure during this manoeuvre leads to a reduction in venous return, thereby underscoring the significance of venous cannulation [12,13].

Aim: The aim of this study was to administer vagus stimulation with the application of standardised cold to the neck area, and thereafter assess the level of pain experienced by patients who underwent venous cannulation on the dorsal side of the hand.

2. Materials and Methods

This single-centre study was conducted within the operating room of Samsun University Training and Research Hospital, Samsun, Turkey) between 18 June and 30 July 2023 following ethics committee approval (Decision no. 11/19 of SÜKAEK-07.06.2023) and Clinical Trials (NCT05920915) registration. Upon their arrival at the operating theatre on the designated day of surgery, patients who had already undergone preoperative preparation for the surgical procedure and administration of anaesthesia were briefed about the aims of the study and informed consent was obtained.

Inclusion Criteria: The study included individuals aged between 18 and 70 years who underwent elective surgery and were classified by the American Society of Anesthesiologists (ASA) as class I-III.

Exclusion Criteria: The study excluded individuals who exhibited the following characteristics: a scar located on the dorsal aspect of the hand, a diagnosis of psoriasis, peripheral vascular disease, chronic analgesic usage, opioid usage, steroid usage, gabapentinoid usage, a history of substance and alcohol use, peripheral neuropathy, ongoing oncological treatment, individuals scheduled for oncological surgery, pregnant women, patients using anti-arrhythmic medication, and patients with limited cooperation.

Randomisation and intervention: Individuals were transported to the preoperative waiting area where they underwent routine monitorisation. The sample size for each group was determined to be 53 patients, with an additional 7 individuals included for potential losses, resulting in a total sample size of 60 individuals for each group. Patients were randomly assigned to three groups: a Control group (Group K), a Cold group (Group M), and a Sham group (Group S). Randomisation was conducted using the Sequentially Numbered, Opaque, Sealed Envelope (SNOSE) technique [14]. Patients whose venous cannulation from the dorsum of the left hand could not be successfully completed in a single attempt were excluded from the study (Figure 1).

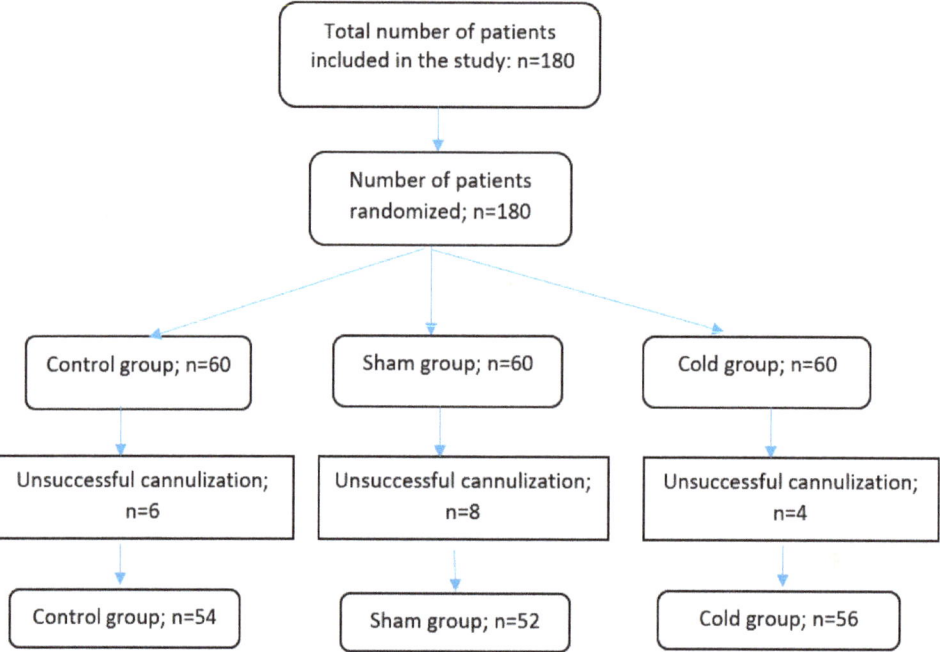

Figure 1. Flow chart of the study. n = number.

Group K (Control group): A waiting period of 30 s was observed prior to opening the vascular access, without any intervention.

Group M (Cold group): Immediately prior to the initiation of vascular access, a marble stone measuring 4 × 5 cm was applied for a duration of 30 s to the carotid artery, specifically positioned 2–3 cm above the collarbone on the sternocleidomastoid muscle (SCM). This marble-derived stone was retrieved from the vegetable shelf of a refrigerator. The stone was subjected to a cooling process at a temperature of −8 °C for a duration of 10 min. Subsequently, the temperature reduced to 11 °C. The temperature of the sample in contact with the palm increases to 12 °C during a span of 1 min and rises to 18 °C over a period of 5 min while placed on a table at room temperature. The marble stone was taken out of the refrigerator at the time of application for each patient and used without waiting.

Group S (Sham group): Prior to initiating vascular access, the bilateral neck region of the patients was prepared by applying a 4 × 5 cm marble stone contained within a polar sheath for a duration of 30 s (Figure 2).

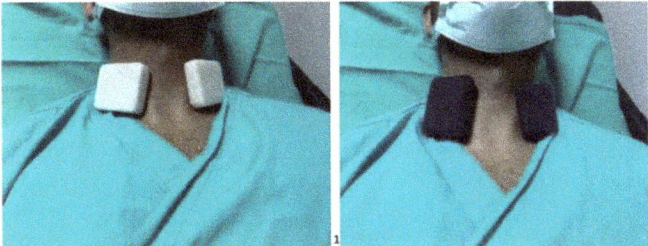

Figure 2. Picture on the left (**1**) is the application of cold marble to the neck area, picture on the right (**2**) is application of non-cold marble to the neck area.

Prior to establishing vascular access, the heart rate (HR), respiratory rate (RR), non-invasive blood pressure (NIBP), and oxygen saturation (SPO2) were measured in all patients. The same parameters were then re-measured following 30 s of contact with a marble stone on the neck area in Group M and Group S. In Group K, the measurements were taken after a 30 s waiting period without any intervention. Subsequently, a single insertion of an 18 gauge (green) intravenous catheter was performed by the same healthcare professional on the dorsal aspect of the left hand. The data of heart rate (HR), respiratory rate (RR), non-invasive blood pressure (NIBP), and peripheral capillary oxygen saturation (SpO2) were promptly documented after the placement of the intravenous catheter. The participants were requested to assess their levels of pain on a scale ranging from 0 to 10 using the numerical pain scale (NRS). The records were recorded by the same nurse blinded to the study.

Statistical Analysis: The data were analysed using the SPSS 21 software. GPower 3.1 was utilised to determine the total sample size required for a study with three groups. The effect size was specified as 0.25, the α error was set at 0.05, and the desired power was 0.80. The computed sample size was found to be 159. The study assessed the NRS scores of three groups and investigated the correlation between heart rate (HR), respiratory rate (RR), and non-invasive blood pressure (NIBP), as well as the oxygen saturation (SPO2) readings of the patients before, immediately after, and following the application of a marble. The normality of distribution was assessed using the Kolmogorov–Smirnov and Shapiro–Wilk tests. The examination of data with a normal distribution involved the utilisation of both the analysis of variance (ANOVA) and the paired samples test. The Kruskal–Wallis, Mann–Whitney U, and Wilcoxon Signed Rank tests were used to analyse data that did not follow a normal distribution. The Chi-square test was conducted by constructing cross tables. Descriptive statistics utilised mean ± standard deviation and percentiles. The results were evaluated using a confidence interval of 95% and a significance level of p 0.05.

3. Results

Data from 162 patients were analysed: 54 in the Control group, 52 in the Sham group, and 56 in the Cold group. The age, gender, and BMI distributions of the patients were comparable between groups (Table 1). No parasympathetic activity-related complications, such as syncope or hypotension, were observed in any of the patients.

Table 1. Demographic data.

		Group			p
		S (n = 52)	K (n = 54)	M (n = 56)	
Age (Mean ± SD)		47.25 ± 17.71	47.3 ± 15.84	44.54 ± 15.56	>0.05
Gender (n)	Male	24	21	24	>0.05
	Female	28	32	32	
BMI (Mean ± SD)		28.71 ± 5.7	28.97 ± 5.44	28.00 ± 5.27	>0.05
ASA (n) I/II/III		7/33/12	5/40/9	18/36/2	

BMI = body mass index; ASA = American Society of Anesthesiologists, SD = standard deviation, n = number.

The initial values for heart rate, respiratory rate, and non-invasive blood pressure were comparable between groups. After vagal stimulation, the mean heart rate in Group M was significantly lower than at baseline ($p < 0.05$). When the initial heart rate values were compared to the heart rate values after vascular access, there was an increase in the heart rate in Groups S and K, while there was a decrease in the heart rate in Group M (Table 2).

Table 2. Changes in heart rates.

	Heart Rate Beats/min (Mean ± SD)		
	Initial Value	**After Vagal Stimulation**	*p*
M (n = 56)	77.07 ± 10.38	72.66 ± 10.29	<0.05
	Initial Value	**After Vascular Access**	
S (n = 52)	74.0 ± 12.56	76.98 ± 14.41	<0.05
K (n = 54)	76.46 ± 12.29	78.04 ± 12.14	>0.05
M (n = 56)	77.07 ± 10.38	76.02 ± 10.43	>0.05

n = number, SD: standard deviation.

When comparing the pain levels of patients undergoing vascular access, the difference between the groups was statistically significant ($p = 0.035$). Significantly reduced NRS values were observed in Group M compared to Group K ($p = 0.038$) and in Group M compared to Group S ($p = 0.048$). When the NRS value of 1–3 was classified as mild pain and 4–10 as moderate to severe pain, significantly more Group M patients experienced mild pain than Group K patients. Table 3 demonstrates that the number of patients with moderate and severe pain was considerably greater in Group K than in Group M ($p = 0.029$).

Table 3. Evaluation of pain scores between groups.

	Groups			*p*
	S (n = 52)	**K (n = 54)**	**M (n = 56)**	
NRS (Mean ± SD)	5.02 ± 2.04	4.94 ± 1.72	[a] 4.16 ± 1.97	<0.05
No Pain (NRS 0)	0	0	1	NA
Mild Pain (NRS 1–3)	14	10	[b] 21	<0.05
Moderate/Severe Pain (NRS 4–10)	38	44	34	>0.05

NRS = numeric rating scale, n = number, SD = standard deviation, NA = Not applicable. [a] $p < 0.05$ when S-K-M, K-M, S-M groups were compared, [b] $p < 0.05$ when M and K groups were compared.

When the respiratory rate and non-invasive blood pressure measurements of the patients were evaluated at baseline, prior to vagal stimulation, after vagal stimulation, and after intravenous access, there was no difference between the groups or within the groups.

4. Discussion and Conclusions

The aim of this study was to evaluate the level of discomfort experienced by individuals undergoing venous cannulation following vagal stimulation induced by the administration of a cold compress to the neck. Our findings indicate that the individuals in Group M, where cold was applied, exhibited less discomfort during vascular access and a better rate of successful vascular access. A notable reduction in the heart rates of the patients in the cold group was noticed in comparison to their initial levels.

Various Valsalva techniques, namely, balloon insufflation, coughing, and breath-holding, are employed for the purpose of stimulating the vagus nerve [12,13,15]. An alternative method of stimulating the vagus nerve involves the application of cold to the cervical region. Jungman previously demonstrated that the application of cold to the neck region results in a reduction in heart rate [7]. In this study, we found that the heart rate of the patients who underwent cold application to the neck region exhibited a statistically significant decrease compared to their initial values. This decrease was seen both immediately after the application of cold and during vascular access. These findings confirm the occurrence of vagal stimulation.

Patients frequently experience discomfort during vascular access, especially when under the stress of a surgical operation. The venous cannulation process is a crucial component of surgical interventions for patients, and successfully navigating this stage without complications brings significant relief. The NRS values observed during vascular access procedures were found to be lower in the group of patients who had undergone cold therapy compared to the other groups. This difference was deemed to be clinically significant, as seen in Table 3. In a study utilising balloon insufflation for vagus stimulation, a substantial proportion of patients reported the absence of any pain, and a much lower number of patients had severe discomfort [12]. Another study demonstrated that patients who underwent plateletpheresis experienced reduced levels of needle insertion pain and anxiety when utilising the Valsalva manoeuvre [15]. In another study, the effect of the Valsalva manoeuvre on the sensation of pain during the insertion of a catheter during spinal anaesthesia was investigated. No patients in the Valsalva group exhibited severe pain, and the proportion of patients who did not report pain was much greater compared to the other groups. In our study, one patient subjected to cold treatment did not report any pain sensation, whereas a total of 21 individuals had mild pain. In their study, Höbek et al. [16] employed the Valsalva manoeuvre as a means to mitigate the vascular access pain experienced by pregnant women. The researchers noted a decrease in pain levels among the participants. The analgesic effect in various clinical scenarios has been investigated in the literature through the utilisation of several approaches to vagus stimulation, such as the Valsalva manoeuvre, stimulation of the vagus nerve from the ear region, and the application of invasive or non-invasive devices targeting the neck region [17,18].

Our research incorporates a novel approach to alleviate venepuncture discomfort by the application of cold stimulation to the vagus nerve. The findings of our investigation indicate that the administration of ice to the vagus nerve has a pain-reducing effect. In the course of our comprehensive literature review, we encountered a dearth of studies investigating the administration of analgesia via vagus nerve stimulation through the application of cold stimuli to the neck area.

This study has several limitations. Firstly, it was conducted in a single centre, which may restrict the generalisability of our findings in other settings. Additionally, the psychological status of the patients, including factors such as anxiety and depression, was not assessed prior to the trial. These psychological factors have been shown to potentially influence pain perception and might have impacted our results. The application of quantifiable markers for assessing nerve vagus stimulation could potentially enhance the effectiveness. An intriguing comparison could be made with a group receiving local anaesthesia.

In conclusion, in this study, we observed that patients whose necks underwent cold compress had a reduced pulse rate that remained low during vascular access. Furthermore, these patients experienced less discomfort during vascular access. The research presented in this study can be regarded as a valuable contribution to the existing body of knowledge on vagus stimulation techniques, which have been employed in several domains such as anxiety management, depression treatment, analgesic efficacy, and epilepsy therapy. To effectively transfer our findings into clinical practice, it is imperative to substantiate our research with studies conducted in diverse contexts such as critical care units, oncology services, and other relevant settings. Additionally, it is crucial to encompass a wide range of age groups, including children and the elderly, to ensure the applicability of our findings across various populations. Furthermore, it is essential to foster broad involvement in these studies to enhance the generalisability and robustness of our conclusions.

Author Contributions: Conceptualization, S.C.A.; Methodology, S.C.A., D.A., G.Ü.Ö., M.S. and İ.O.; Formal analysis, S.C.A.; Investigation, S.C.A. and A.Ç.; Resources, S.C.A.; Data curation, S.C.A., H.B.A. and A.Ç.; Writing—original draft, S.C.A. All authors have read and agreed to the published version of the manuscript.

Funding: This research received no external funding.

Institutional Review Board Statement: Our study was carried out in accordance with the principles of the Declaration of Helsinki, with the approval of Samsun University Clinical Research Ethics Committee (Samsun, Turkey) dated 11/19 of SÜKAEK-07.06.2023.

Informed Consent Statement: Informed consent was obtained from all subjects participating in the study.

Data Availability Statement: The corresponding author can share data whenever desired.

Conflicts of Interest: The authors declare no conflict of interest.

References

1. Butt, M.F.; Albusoda, A.; Farmer, A.D.; Aziz, Q. The anatomical basis for transcutaneous auricular vagus nerve stimulation. *J. Anat.* **2020**, *236*, 588–611. [CrossRef] [PubMed]
2. Courties, A.; Berenbaum, F.; Sellam, J. Vagus nerve stimulation in musculoskeletal diseases. *Jt. Bone Spine* **2021**, *88*, 105149. [CrossRef] [PubMed]
3. Asher, G.N.; Jonas, D.E.; Coeytaux, R.R.; Reilly, A.C.; Loh, Y.L.; Motsinger-Reif, A.A.; Winham, S.J. Auriculotherapy for pain management: A systematic review and meta-analysis of randomized controlled trials. *J. Altern. Complement. Med.* **2010**, *16*, 1097–1108. [CrossRef] [PubMed]
4. Hilz, M.J. Transcutaneous vagus nerve stimulation—A brief introduction and overview. *Auton. Neurosci.* **2022**, *243*, 103038. [CrossRef] [PubMed]
5. Yap, J.Y.; Keatch, C.; Lambert, E.; Woods, W.; Stoddart, P.R.; Kameneva, T. Critical review of transcutaneous vagus nerve stimulation: Challenges for translation to clinical practice. *Front. Neurosci.* **2020**, *14*, 284. [CrossRef] [PubMed]
6. Kumar, S.; Gautam, S.K.S.; Gupta, D.; Agarwal, A.; Dhirraj, S.; Khuba, S. The effect of Valsalva maneuver in attenuating skin puncture pain during spinal anesthesia: A randomized controlled trial. *Korean J. Anesthesiol.* **2016**, *69*, 27–31. [CrossRef] [PubMed]
7. Jungmann, M.; Vencatachellum, S.; Van Ryckeghem, D.; Vögele, C. Effects of cold stimulation on cardiac-vagal activation in healthy participants: Randomized controlled trial. *JMIR Form. Res.* **2018**, *2*, e10257. [CrossRef] [PubMed]
8. Agarwal, A.; Sinha, P.K.; Tandon, M.; Dhiraaj, S.; Singh, U. Evaluating the efficacy of the valsalva maneuver on venous cannulation pain: A prospective, randomized study. *Anesth. Analg.* **2005**, *101*, 1230–1232. [CrossRef] [PubMed]
9. Öztürk, E.; Erdil, F.A.; Begeç, Z.; Yücel, A.; Şanli, M.; Ersoy, M.Ö. İntravenöz kanülasyon ağrısına buzun etkisi. *Fırat Tıp Derg.* **2009**, *14*, 108–110.
10. Fields, J.M.; Piela, N.E.; Ku, B.S. Association between Multiple IV attempts and Perceived Pain levels in the Emergency Department. *J. Vasc. Access* **2014**, *15*, 514–518. [CrossRef] [PubMed]
11. Fathi, M.; Izanloo, A.; Jahanbakhsh, S.; Gilani, M.T.; Majidzadeh, A.; Benhangi, A.S.; Paravi, N. Central Venous Cannulation of the Internal Jugular Vein Using Ultrasound-Guided and Anatomical Landmark Techniques. *Anesth. Pain Med.* **2016**, *6*, e35803. [CrossRef] [PubMed]
12. Gupta, D.; Agarwal, A.; Dhiraaj, S.; Tandon, M.; Kumar, M.; Singh, R.S.; Singh, P.K.; Singh, U. An evaluation of efficacy of balloon inflation on venous cannulation pain in children: A prospective, randomized, controlled study. *Anesth. Analg.* **2006**, *102*, 1372–1375. [CrossRef] [PubMed]
13. Paccione, C.E.; Stubhaug, A.; Diep, L.M.; Rosseland, L.A.; Jacobsen, H.B. Meditative-based diaphragmatic breathing vs. vagus nerve stimulation in the treatment of fibromyalgia—A randomized controlled trial: Body vs. machine. *Front. Neurol.* **2022**, *13*, 1030927. [CrossRef] [PubMed]
14. Doig, G.S.; Simpson, F. Randomization and allocation concealment: A practical guide for researchers. *J. Crit. Care* **2005**, *20*, 187–191. [CrossRef] [PubMed]
15. Srivastava, A.; Kumar, S.; Agarwal, A.; Khetan, D.; Katharia, R.; Mishra, P.; Khati, S.; Gautam, S.; Sandeep, K. Evaluation of efficacy of Valsalva for attenuating needle puncture pain in first time nonremunerated voluntary plateletpheresis donors: A prospective, randomized controlled trial. *Asian J. Transfus. Sci.* **2021**, *15*, 68. [CrossRef] [PubMed]
16. Akarsu, R.H.; Kuş, B.; Akarsu, G.D. Effects of valsalva maneuver, emla cream, and stress ball for pregnant women's venipuncture pain. *Altern. Ther. Health Med.* **2021**, *27*, 108–114.

17. Széles, J.; Kampusch, S.; Le, V.; Enajat, D.; Kaniusas, E.; Neumayer, C. Clinical Effectiveness of Percutaneous Auricular Vagus Nerve Stimulation in Chronic Back Pain Patients—A Single-Centre Retrospective Analysis. *Ann. Pain Med.* **2021**, *3*, 1009.
18. Patel, A.B.; Bibawy, P.P.; Majeed, Z.; Gan, W.L.; Ackland, G.L. Trans-auricular vagus nerve stimulation to reduce perioperative pain and morbidity: Protocol for a single-blind analyser-masked randomised controlled trial. *BJA Open* **2022**, *2*, 100017. [CrossRef] [PubMed]

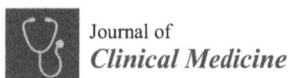

Article

Severe Postoperative Pain in Total Knee Arthroplasty Patients: Risk Factors, Insights and Implications for Pain Management via a Digital Health Approach

Julien Lebleu [1,*], Andries Pauwels [1], Hervé Poilvache [2], Philippe Anract [3] and Anissa Belbachir [4]

1   moveUP, Cantersteen 47, 1000 Brussels, Belgium
2   Orthopedic Surgery Department, CHIREC, 1420 Braine-l'Alleud, Belgium
3   Service de Chirurgie Orthopédique, Hopital Cochin, Université Paris Cité, 75014 Paris, France
4   Service d'Anesthésie, Réanimation et Médecine Périopératoire, Hopital Cochin, Université Paris Cité, 75014 Paris, France
*   Correspondence: julien@moveup.care

Abstract: Up to 25% of patients undergoing knee arthroplasty report chronic pain postoperatively. Early identification of high-risk individuals can enhance pain management strategies. This retrospective analysis investigates the incidence of severe postoperative pain and its associated risk factors among 740 patients who underwent total knee arthroplasty. Utilizing a digital application, patients provided comprehensive data encompassing pre- and postoperative pain levels, analgesic usage, and completed a chronic pain risk assessment. Participants were categorized into two distinct groups based on their pain status at three months post-op: Group D+ (14%), characterized by pain scores exceeding 40/100 and/or the utilization of level 2 or 3 analgesics, and Group D− (86%), who did not meet these criteria. An analysis of pain trajectories within these groups revealed a non-linear progression, with specific patterns emerging amongst those predisposed to chronic pain. Notably, patients with a trajectory towards chronic pain exhibited a plateau in pain intensity approximately three weeks post-surgery. Significant preoperative risk factors were identified, including elevated initial pain levels, the presence of comorbidities, pain in other body areas, heightened joint sensitivity and stiffness. This study highlights the utility of digital platforms in enhancing patient care, particularly through the continuous monitoring of pain. Such an approach facilitates the early identification of potential complications and enables timely interventions.

Keywords: knee surgery; chronic pain; mhealth; analgesia; pain trajectory; pain management; prehabilitation

Citation: Lebleu, J.; Pauwels, A.; Poilvache, H.; Anract, P.; Belbachir, A. Severe Postoperative Pain in Total Knee Arthroplasty Patients: Risk Factors, Insights and Implications for Pain Management via a Digital Health Approach. *J. Clin. Med.* **2023**, *12*, 7695. https://doi.org/10.3390/jcm12247695

Academic Editors: Felice Eugenio Agro, Giuseppe Pascarella and Fabio Costa

Received: 26 October 2023
Revised: 8 December 2023
Accepted: 11 December 2023
Published: 15 December 2023

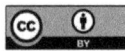
1. Introduction

Despite the implementation of multimodal pain management techniques, the postoperative phase following total knee arthroplasty (TKA) frequently results in significant pain for patients. This often leads to adverse patient outcomes, including dissatisfaction, prolonged hospitalization, diminished quality of life, and non-adherence to rehabilitation protocols [1]. Additionally, the extended use of analgesics can precipitate adverse side effects [2], contributing to the development of chronic pain symptoms in 10 to 30% of cases [3,4].

The current understanding of the risk factors contributing to chronic pain post-TKA is incomplete, despite extensive research efforts [5,6]. Research has identified several potential risk factors, including local inflammation due to surgery, nerve sensitization, psychological factors such as anxiety and depression, pain catastrophizing, and preoperative opioid use [7–10]. Accurately predicting which patients will develop chronic pain remains a significant challenge. However, recent studies have highlighted the potential of perioperative pain patterns as a valuable indicator for identifying patients at risk of chronic pain [11–13].

The past decade has seen the advent of digital health technologies enabling the continuous collection of perioperative data [14–17], including pain scores [18].

This development has provided physicians with enhanced insights into patient pain experiences, thereby improving pain management strategies. By integrating these technologies with the knowledge of identified risk factors, there is potential for a more profound understanding and prediction of chronic pain post-TKA [19,20].

This study aims to: (1) characterize the structure of acute pain trajectories during the postoperative period following TKA using a digital platform, (2) investigate risk factors potentially leading to chronic pain, and (3) examine the differences in recovery patterns among patients who develop chronic pain.

2. Materials and Methods

2.1. Study Design and Data Source

We conducted a retrospective observational study using anonymized depersonalized data from the database of moveUP digital therapies (moveUP solution, Brussels, Belgium). The database comprises data from patients who underwent hip and knee arthroplasty across Belgium, France, and the Netherlands. A cohort of 740 patients who underwent elective total knee arthroplasty was selected, covering the period from November 2017 to June 2023. Patients were included in the study if they used the digital application for at least 70 days after surgery and completed their patient reported outcome measures at 3 months postop. Prior to the inclusion, each patient provided written informed consent for the scientific use of their anonymized data. Regulatory guidelines were followed with no involvement of institutional review board (IRB) approval as this study used anonymized patient-level data.

2.2. Data Collection System

All data collection was facilitated via the moveUP® application (moveUP®, Brussels, Belgium), which is registered as a medical device. This application operates on a smart virtual platform designed for digital monitoring, utilizing both objective and subjective patient data. The platform consists of two main components: a patient-facing mobile application and a web-based dashboard utilized by the care provider.

In concurrence with data collection, the application provided patients with timely educational materials regarding their postoperative recovery. These informational resources were developed and validated in collaboration with hospital care teams [14], ensuring the delivery of credible and accurate guidance to facilitate patient recovery (Figure 1).

2.3. Outcomes

The patients used the moveUP app to collect pre- and postoperative pain data, chronic pain risk factors, analgesic usage and physical activity (using a commercial activity tracker (Garmin Vivofit 4) worn 24/7 by the patients.). Pain and swelling were assessed daily using a visual analog scale (VAS: 0–100 scale, higher score indicating worse pain) [21]. Pain medication type and frequency was also assessed daily (level 1, 2 and 3 painkillers).

Potential chronic pain risk factors were collected pre-operatively: age, gender, body mass index (BMI), type and number of comorbidities, patient reported sensitivity, patient reported stiffness, preoperative pain intensity at rest, preoperative pain intensity at night, and presence of pain elsewhere at multiple sites (Table 1). Patient-reported outcomes such as Knee Osteoarthritis Outcome score (KOOS), and EuroQol 5-Dimension (EQ5D) were measured before surgery and 6 weeks, 3 months, 6 months, 1 and 2 years after surgery through the app.

2.4. Chronic Pain

The International Association for the Study of Pain (IASP) defines chronic post-surgical pain as pain that persists beyond the healing process, i.e., at least three months after surgery [22]. Patients were divided into two groups: those exhibiting pain scores greater than 40/100 and/or consuming level 2 or 3 analgesics were categorized as D+, and those who did not fulfill these criteria at three months post-surgery were categorized as D− [23].

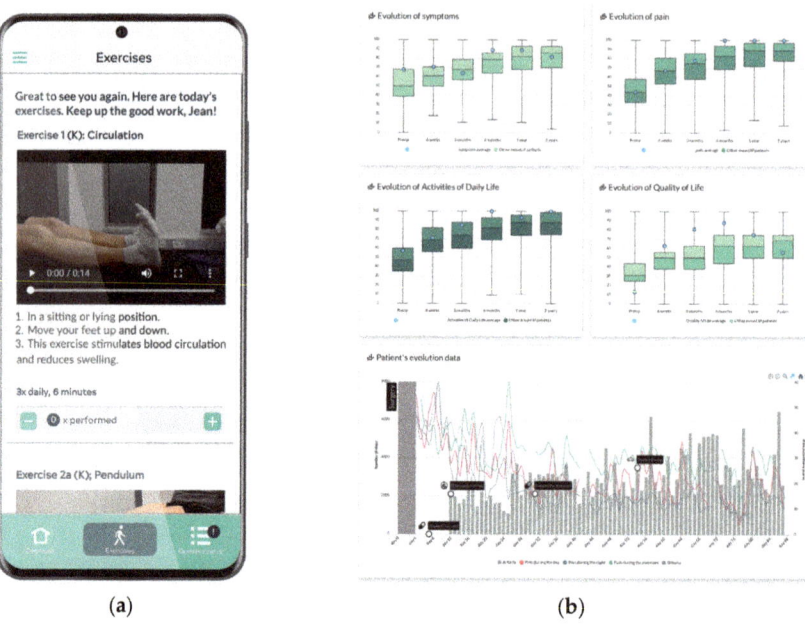

(a)   (b)

Figure 1. Patient application (**a**) and example of an evolution report showing patient reported outcomes scores against a population and the evolution of daily data (**b**).

Table 1. Questions asked through the application.

Questions	Answer Options
Indicate on the slider the stiffness you experienced in your joint?	0–100 slider—none—very stiff
What is the intensity of your pain?	0–100 slider—no pain—intolerable pain
Does your affected joint feel swollen? (no swelling—very swollen)	0–100 slider—no swelling—very swollen
In the last 7 days, how bad was you pain at rest?	0–100 slider—no pain—worst pain imaginable
In the last 7 days, how bad was your pain at night?	0–100 slider—no pain—worst pain imaginable
On a scale from 0 to 10, how severe is the sensitivity in/around the joint?	0–10 choice—normal- not sensitive at all, extremely sensitive
Do you experience complaints to other areas surrounding your index joint?	Yes—No
Did you take any medication today?	Yes—No
Add the medication you took today below (painkillers, anti-inflammatory, anti-coagulants, etc.)	Multiple choice + free entry

2.5. Statistical Analysis

Descriptive statistics were used to describe the data with median (interquartile range) for continuous variables, and number (percentage) for categorical variables. The Chi-square test was applied to assess proportional differences between groups. The Mann–Whitney U test was utilized to compare the parameters between the groups, with an alpha error threshold set at 0.05.

3. Results

Demographic characteristics of the study participants are delineated in Table 2. Within the cohort, the non-chronic pain group (D−) constituted 632 patients (85%), whereas the chronic pain group (D+) comprised 108 patients (15%). At the three-month postoperative interval, 89 patients reported a pain intensity exceeding 40/100, and 19 patients were using level 2 or 3 analgesics. The majority of participants in both cohorts were retired. A higher proportion of females was observed in the chronic pain group (71%) compared to the non-chronic pain group (56%).

Table 2. Demographics comparison between chronic and non-chronic pain groups.

Characteristic	Chronic Pain (D+)	Non-Chronic (D−)	*p*-Value
N (%)	108 (14.6%)	632 (85.4%)	/
Age (years), median (IQR)	61.0 (56.0–70.0)	63.0 (57.0–69.0)	0.989
BMI, median (IQR)	29.0 (26.1–32.6)	29.0 (26.1–32.7)	0.711
Gender, N (%)			0.007
Female	77 (71)	352 (56)	
Male	31 (29)	273 (43)	
Unknown	0	7 (1)	
Employment status, N (%)			0.034
Employed	1 (1)	43 (8)	
Unemployed	88 (98)	497 (92)	
Educational background, N (%)			0.253
Primary school	11 (12)	48 (9)	
Secondary school	47 (52)	260 (48)	
Bachelor degree	20 (22)	139 (26)	
Master degree	9 (10)	88 (16)	
I prefer not to answer this question	2 (2)	4 (1)	

N: number of patients, IQR: interquartile range.

Preoperative pain intensity was reported to be greater during the daytime as opposed to nighttime (Figure 2). A notable peak in pain was recorded within the initial two days post-surgery, which then subsided by the third day and approached a plateau around day 45.

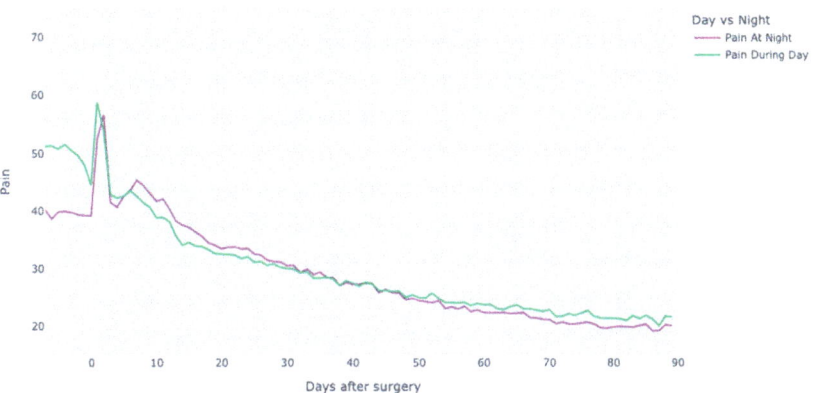

Figure 2. Pain intensity evolution during day and night over the 90 days post-surgery for the whole TKA population.

During the first and second weeks post-surgery, the chronic pain cohort consistently reported elevated pain levels relative to the non-chronic pain cohort, with these disparities proving to be statistically significant. Over time, the divergence in pain trajectories became more pronounced (Figure 3). The pain levels in the chronic pain cohort began to plateau after three weeks, while those in the non-chronic pain cohort continued on a declining trend.

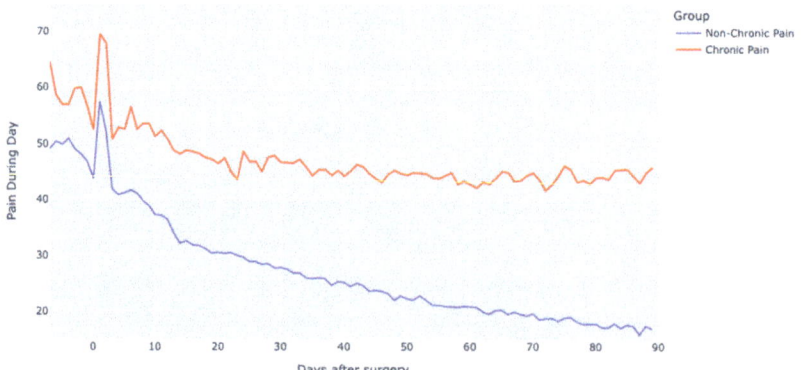

Figure 3. Pain experienced during the day for the chronic and non-chronic pain group. Rel to surgery: relative to surgery.

Comparative analysis revealed significant statistical differences across most measured parameters between the chronic pain group (D+) and the non-chronic pain group (D−) as presented in Table 3. Patients in the chronic pain cohort were more likely to have at least one comorbidity, with 79% of them reporting such conditions.

Table 3. Risk factors comparison between chronic and non-chronic pain groups.

Characteristic	Chronic Pain (D+)	Non-Chronic (D−)	*p*-Value
Number of comorbidities, %			<0.001
0	21	53	
1	57	31	
>2	22	16	
Pre-operative parameters			
Number of patients with pain elsewhere than surgical site, %	60	42	
Percentage of patients in each pain category, %			<0.001
No pain—VAS 0–4	0	1	
Mild pain—VAS 5–44	17	42	
Moderate pain- VAS 45–74	70	55	
Severe pain—VAS 75–100	13	2	
Sensitivity (0/10) (median, IQR)	8.0 (7.0–8.0)	7.0 (6.0–8.0)	0.002
Stiffness (0/100) (median, IQR)	59.3 (49.3–73.0)	46.2 (31.6–59.8)	<0.001
Pain at night (0/100) (median, IQR)	52.8 (41.0–63.4)	36.7 (22.7–51.3)	<0.001
Swelling (0/100) (median, IQR)	29.8 (12.9–53.6)	25.0 (11.4–50.7)	0.40
Physical activity (number of steps) (median, IQR)	3637 (2545–5490)	3916 (2262–5931)	0.75
Peri-operative parameters	Chronic pain (D+)	Non-Chronic (D−)	
Pain first week (0/100) (median, IQR)	52.6 (43.4–62.7)	37.6 (27.7–47.4)	<0.001
Pain second week (0/100) (median, IQR)	48.1 (41.2–56.8)	31.2 (22.6–41.4)	<0.001
Patient reported outcomes	Chronic pain (D+)	Non-Chronic (D−)	

Table 3. *Cont.*

Characteristic	Chronic Pain (D+)	Non-Chronic (D−)	*p*-Value
EQ5D (VAS score) (median, IQR)	54.0 (38.0–72.0)	62.0 (43.0–76.0)	0.009
KOOS Pain (median, IQR)	39.0 (31.0–50.0)	47.0 (36.0–58.0)	<0.001
KOOS Symptoms (median, IQR)	50.0 (39.0–64.0)	54.0 (43.0–68.0)	0.47
KOOS Activities of Daily Life (median, IQR)	40.5 (31.8–51.5)	50.0 (39.5–63.0)	<0.001
KOOS Quality of Life (median, IQR)	19.0 (6.0–31.0)	25.0 (19.0–38.0)	<0.001

N: number of patients, IQR: interquartile range, VAS: visual analogic scale.

Furthermore, a substantial proportion of the chronic pain group reported experiencing pain in areas other than the surgical site (60% in D+ vs. 42% in D−). This group also demonstrated statistically significant higher levels of sensitivity, stiffness, and pain at night (*p*-value < 0.05). A higher proportion of the chronic pain group experienced moderate and severe pain than the non-chronic pain group [24].

When considering preoperative patient-reported outcome measures, those with chronic pain showed significantly lower scores, particularly in KOOS Pain, KOOS Activities of Daily Life, and KOOS Quality of Life domains (*p*-value < 0.05).

Postoperatively, the chronic pain group consistently scored lower across all KOOS subscales when compared to their counterparts without chronic pain (*p* < 0.05), except for the KOOS Symptoms domain, which only diverged at 6 months, and one and two years post-surgery (*p* < 0.05), as indicated in Figure 4.

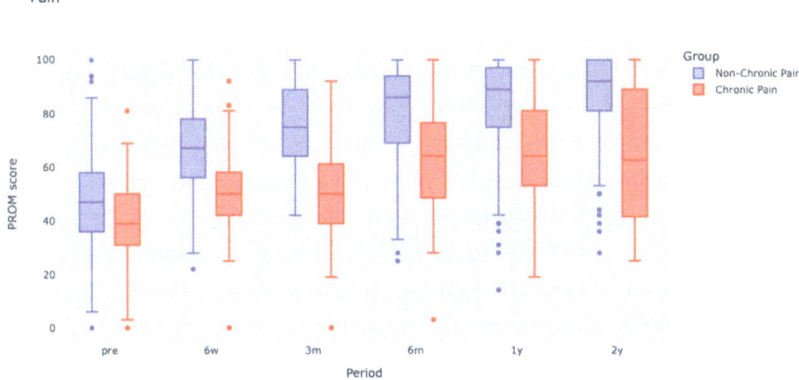

Figure 4. Box plots illustrating the distribution of KOOS pain in chronic and non-chronic pain groups over a 2-year duration. PROM: Patient reported outcome score for KOOS pain.

Preoperative physical activity levels, approximating 5000 steps/day, were comparable between the groups. Any differences in early postoperative physical activity were minimal, but tended to grow over time (Figure 5). Similarly, patient-reported swelling showed no preoperative variance but escalated as time progressed (Figure 6). The duration of NSAID use differed between the groups; patients with chronic pain used NSAIDs for a median of 51 days (IQR 31–76 days), while those without chronic pain had a shorter duration of 33 days (IQR 21–58 days).

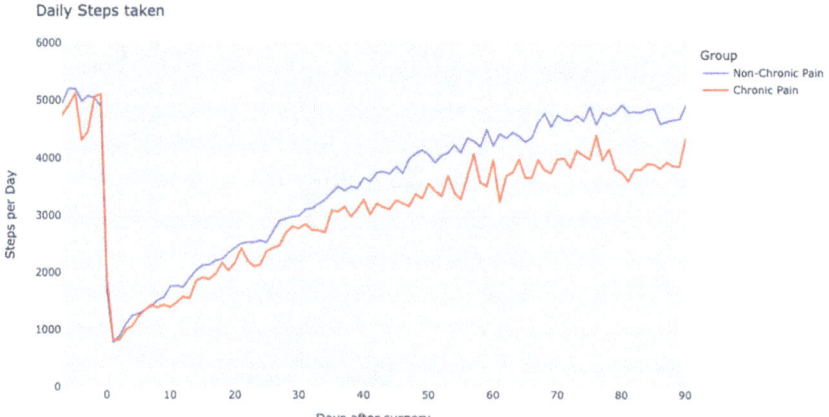

Figure 5. Recovery of physical activity level (number of steps/day) in chronic and non-chronic pain groups. Rel to surgery: relative to surgery.

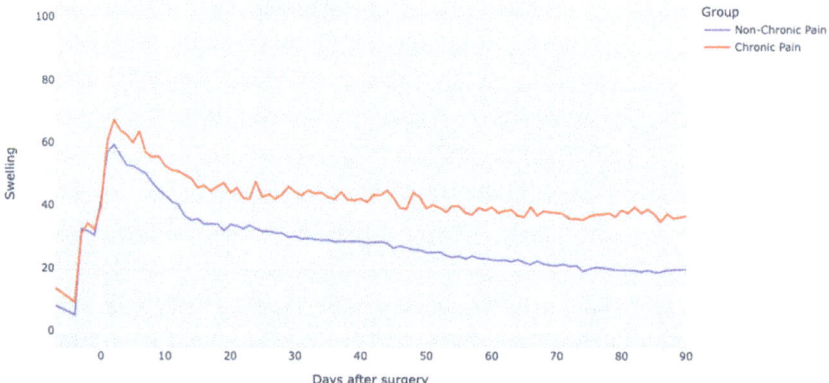

Figure 6. Patient reported swelling (VAS scale 0–100) in chronic and non-chronic pain groups. Rel to surgery: relative to surgery.

4. Discussion

The primary objectives of our investigation were to: (1) characterize the structure of acute pain trajectories post-surgery, (2) identify risk factors potentially leading to chronic pain, and (3) assess recovery patterns in patients with chronic pain post-TKA.

The concept of pain trajectories is a relatively recent development, distinct from the traditional approach of assessing pain at discrete time points [11]. Pain does not follow a linear progression over the 90 days following surgery; instead, it tends to follow a distinct pattern [25]. After surgery, there is an acute pain phase as a reaction to the surgical trauma, followed by an early recovery around day 3 with a gradual reduction in the peak pain. Subsequently, the pain continues to decrease gradually, eventually reaching a plateau that many patients describe as a manageable level of pain. However, it is important to note that not all patients follow this pattern, and some require specific attention. The transition from subacute to chronic pain is of significant research interest. In the Althaus study [11], pain resolution at 5 days in one of the patient groups did not occur despite analgesic treatment. Previous analyses suggest that psycho-social variables such as depression and anxiety may play a role in pain resolution by influencing degree of support [26].

By dividing the population into two groups, we gained a better understanding of the typical pain progression for patients who ultimately experience chronic pain. Notably, these patients deviated from the expected pattern of diminishing pain intensity, instead reaching a plateau in pain levels by the third postoperative week. Furthermore, this unfavorable trajectory is reflected in worse KOOS pain scores at 2 years post-surgery. The total knee arthroplasty (TKA) population is inherently diverse, and this arbitrary binary classification underscores the necessity for personalized, person-centered care.

The link between high preoperative pain intensity and the evolution of chronic pain postoperatively was reinforced, with our chronic pain cohort exhibiting elevated initial pain levels [5,6]. This suggests a heightened nociceptive response or an increased sensitivity of the pain signaling system. Nevertheless, the marginal differences in initial pain between the groups preclude its utility as a standalone prognostic marker. In contrast, the divergence in pain levels at two and three weeks postoperative offers a more definitive prognostic indicator, signaling an optimal period for clinical intervention. Four studies already investigated the association between pain severity during the first two weeks and chronic pain, but there is insufficient evidence to draw firm conclusion [27]. The question remains about why these two groups exhibit such divergent pain resolution trajectories.

The study confirmed that having pain in multiple areas or other health issues increases the risk of chronic pain post-TKA, which aligns with previous research [4–6]. Predictive models using simple risk factors show promise in identifying patients at risk for chronic pain [28]. Yet, this study did not capture data on neuropathic pain or psychological factors like pain catastrophizing, depression, and anxiety, which are known to affect pain perception and recovery [29].

We split the TKA patients into groups based on pain at the three-month mark, because the IASP identifies this as when acute pain may become chronic. Our analysis shows it is unnecessary to wait six months to see if a patient's recovery is off track. Most improvement happens in the first three months post-surgery [30,31], and higher pain scores at three months could indicate worse outcomes at one and two years. Singh et al. observed similar patterns, with distinct pain trajectories at eight weeks predicting six-month outcomes [13]. While most patients recover typically, some have different experiences up to eight years post-surgery [32].

Our chronic pain incidence was 14%, lower than the 30% found in some studies [23]. Ongoing pain tracking could help clinicians spot problems and tailor treatments. Digital tools are already making strides in patient education, reducing post-TKA pain [16]. A stronger digital link between patients and care providers, including automatic alerts for quick response by pain management teams, might further cut chronic pain rates in a cost-effective manner.

Unfortunately, information regarding the type of anesthesia used in the 40 different centers was not available. While the specific anesthesia details may enhance the granularity of our analysis, we contend that the scale and diversity of our dataset allow for valuable insights into broader trends and practices. However, as regional anesthesia techniques, such as epidural anesthesia [33] and fascial plane blocks [34], have been employed to alleviate acute pain after TKA, this may limit the generalizability of our study. Indeed, while these techniques primarily target perioperative pain, there is evidence suggesting that effective pain control during the immediate postoperative period may have implications for the development of chronic pain [33–36]. The potential mechanisms underlying the observed reduction in chronic pain incidence involve the prevention of central sensitization and modulation of the inflammatory response. Regional anesthesia techniques, by targeting specific nerve pathways, may contribute to a more controlled perioperative pain environment, mitigating the neuroplastic changes associated with chronic pain development [37]. Furthermore, the attenuation of the inflammatory response during the early stages of recovery may have implications for long-term pain outcomes [38].

Pain is linked to swelling in the acute phase, which is influenced by how active patients are [39]. To manage this, patients received custom advice from physical therapists. They used standard inflammation control like ice, activity management, and NSAIDs. These approaches may affect pain over time. Despite measures to control inflammation, the chronic pain group still showed more swelling by a score of 20/100 at three months post-surgery compared to their counterparts. The impact of these interventions is more visible on an individual level, as illustrated by a case where a patient's early resumption of physical activity led to stagnant pain and swelling levels. Following the advice to significantly reduce physical activity after the first consultation, the patient experienced a decrease in pain after a few weeks. While instructive, more research is needed to clarify the influence of activity pacing and NSAID use on postoperative swelling and pain (Figure 7).

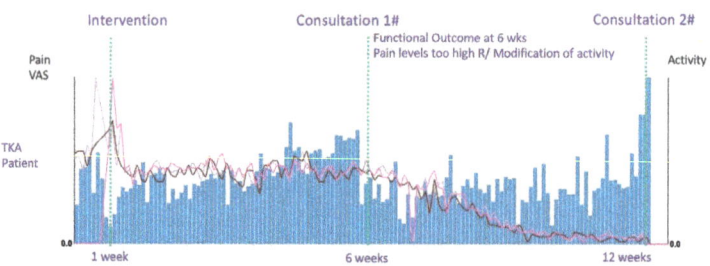

Figure 7. Patient case. Blue bars represent the level of physical activity. The lines represent the pain and the swelling.

The study has several limitations. Its retrospective design can show associations but not causality. Prospective studies are necessary to understand the cause-anD−effect relationship between risk factors and chronic pain. The selection of participants may also introduce bias, as it relies on patients consistently using a mobile app for data collection, potentially excluding those who recovered quickly or did not use the app. Additionally, while the study points to pre-surgery risk factors for chronic pain, it may not account for all variables that could affect pain outcomes. The study also did not differentiate between the specific causes of chronic pain, such as extra-articular or intra-articular issues [40], which might influence results and introduce confounders. Further research is required to parse out these distinctions for a clearer understanding of chronic pain development after TKA.

5. Conclusions

In this research, we conducted a detailed examination of acute pain trajectories post-total knee arthroplasty (TKA) and investigated the risk factors for chronic pain. Our results bring to light the complex nature of postoperative pain, stressing the critical role of early detection and individualized management strategies in optimizing outcomes for TKA patients.

The analysis indicated that pain after TKA does not follow a simple, linear decline, but rather presents in various patterns, particularly a plateauing of pain levels after the third week in patients who develop chronic pain. This suggests the necessity for adaptive care plans that are responsive to the unique pain experiences of each patient.

Identified preoperative risk factors for chronic pain included not only high pain levels before surgery, but also the presence of multiple comorbidities, pain in other body areas, increased sensitivity, joint stiffness, and nocturnal pain. These findings are instrumental in forming predictive models that can be used to anticipate chronic pain and customize early interventions.

The study highlights the efficacy of continuous pain monitoring with digital platforms in enhancing patient care. By establishing a digital interface between patients and healthcare providers, there is an opportunity for more immediate detection of complications and the provision of prompt care, which may lead to a decrease in the occurrence of chronic pain.

To conclude, this study advances our understanding of the postoperative pain landscape and the elements that influence chronic pain after TKA. Emphasizing personalized and interdisciplinary approaches, and incorporating digital healthcare tools, this research points towards improved patient outcomes and the elevation of care standards in the field

J. Clin. Med. **2023**, *12*, 7695

of orthopedic surgery. The insights gained herein pave the way for future research to refine clinical approaches in managing post-TKA pain.

Author Contributions: Conceptualization, J.L., A.P. and A.B.; methodology, J.L., A.P. and A.B.; software, A.P.; validation, J.L., A.P. and A.B.; formal analysis, J.L. and A.P.; investigation, J.L, A.P. and A.B.; resources, J.L.; data curation, J.L. and A.P.; writing—original draft preparation, J.L., A.P. and A.B.; writing—review and editing, J.L., A.P., P.A., H.P. and A.B.; visualization, J.L. and A.P.; supervision, P.A. and A.B.; project administration, J.L. All authors have read and agreed to the published version of the manuscript.

Funding: This research received no external funding.

Institutional Review Board Statement: Regulatory guidelines were followed with no involvement of institutional review board (IRB) approval as this study used anonymized patient-level data.

Informed Consent Statement: Informed consent was obtained from all subjects involved in the study.

Data Availability Statement: The data presented in this study are available on request from the corresponding author. The data are not publicly available due to privacy reasons.

Acknowledgments: We thank Christian Bobak for English language editing.

Conflicts of Interest: Julien Lebleu is an employee of the company who build the software used to collect data Andries Pauwels is an employee of the company who build the software used to collect data. Philippe Anract, Anissa Belbachir and Hervé Poilvache have no conflicts of interest to declare.

References

1. Gan, T.J. Poorly Controlled Postoperative Pain: Prevalence, Consequences, and Prevention. *J. Pain Res.* **2017**, *10*, 2287–2298. [CrossRef]
2. Fuzier, R.; Rousset, J.; Bataille, B.; Salces-y-Nédéo, A.; Maguès, J.-P. One Half of Patients Reports Persistent Pain Three Months after Orthopaedic Surgery. *Anaesth. Crit. Care Pain Med.* **2015**, *34*, 159–164. [CrossRef]
3. Beswick, A.D.; Wylde, V.; Gooberman-Hill, R.; Blom, A.; Dieppe, P. What Proportion of Patients Report Long-Term Pain after Total Hip or Knee Replacement for Osteoarthritis? A Systematic Review of Prospective Studies in Unselected Patients. *BMJ Open* **2012**, *2*, e000435. [CrossRef]
4. Wylde, V.; Beswick, A.; Bruce, J.; Blom, A.; Howells, N.; Gooberman-Hill, R. Chronic Pain after Total Knee Arthroplasty. *EFORT Open Rev.* **2018**, *3*, 461–470. [CrossRef] [PubMed]
5. Ashoorion, V.; Sadeghirad, B.; Wang, L.; Noori, A.; Abdar, M.; Kim, Y.; Chang, Y.; Rehman, N.; Lopes, L.C.; Couban, R.J.; et al. Predictors of Persistent Post-Surgical Pain Following Total Knee Arthroplasty: A Systematic Review and Meta-Analysis of Observational Studies. *Pain Med.* **2023**, *24*, 369–381. [CrossRef] [PubMed]
6. Lewis, G.N.; Rice, D.A.; McNair, P.J.; Kluger, M. Predictors of Persistent Pain after Total Knee Arthroplasty: A Systematic Review and Meta-Analysis. *Br. J. Anaesth.* **2015**, *114*, 551–561. [CrossRef]
7. Priol, R.; Pasquier, G.; Putman, S.; Migaud, H.; Dartus, J.; Wattier, J.-M. Trajectory of Chronic and Neuropathic Pain, Anxiety and Depressive Symptoms and Pain Catastrophizing after Total Knee Replacement. Results of a Prospective, Single-Center Study at a Mean Follow-up of 7.5 Years. *Orthop. Traumatol. Surg. Res.* **2023**, *109*, 103543. [CrossRef]
8. Kunkel, S.T.; Gregory, J.J.; Sabatino, M.J.; Borsinger, T.M.; Fillingham, Y.A.; Jevsevar, D.S.; Moschetti, W.E. Does Preoperative Opioid Consumption Increase the Risk of Chronic Postoperative Opioid Use After Total Joint Arthroplasty? *Arthroplast. Today* **2021**, *10*, 46–50. [CrossRef]
9. Fletcher, D.; Stamer, U.M.; Pogatzki-Zahn, E.; Zaslansky, R.; Tanase, N.V.; Perruchoud, C.; Kranke, P.; Komann, M.; Lehman, T.; Meissner, W.; et al. Chronic Postsurgical Pain in Europe: An Observational Study. *Eur. J. Anaesthesiol. EJA* **2015**, *32*, 725–734. [CrossRef] [PubMed]
10. Li, C.Y.; Ng Cheong Chung, K.J.; Ali, O.M.E.; Chung, N.D.H.; Li, C.H. Literature Review of the Causes of Pain Following Total Knee Replacement Surgery: Prosthesis, Inflammation and Arthrofibrosis. *EFORT Open Rev.* **2020**, *5*, 534–543. [CrossRef]
11. Althaus, A.; Arránz Becker, O.; Moser, K.-H.; Lux, E.A.; Weber, F.; Neugebauer, E.; Simanski, C. Postoperative Pain Trajectories and Pain Chronification—An Empirical Typology of Pain Patients. *Pain Med.* **2018**, *19*, 2536–2545. [CrossRef] [PubMed]
12. Chapman, C.R.; Donaldson, G.W.; Davis, J.J.; Bradshaw, D.H. Improving Individual Measurement of Postoperative Pain: The Pain Trajectory. *J. Pain* **2011**, *12*, 257–262. [CrossRef] [PubMed]
13. Singh, J.A.; Lemay, C.A.; Nobel, L.; Yang, W.; Weissman, N.; Saag, K.G.; Allison, J.; Franklin, P.D. Association of Early Postoperative Pain Trajectories with Longer-Term Pain Outcome after Primary Total Knee Arthroplasty. *JAMA Netw. Open* **2019**, *2*, e1915105. [CrossRef] [PubMed]

14. Lebleu, J.; Pauwels, A.; Anract, P.; Parratte, S.; Van Overschelde, P.; Van Onsem, S. Digital Rehabilitation after Knee Arthroplasty: A Multi-Center Prospective Longitudinal Cohort Study. *J. Pers. Med.* **2023**, *13*, 824. [CrossRef] [PubMed]

15. van der Meij, E.; Bouwsma, E.V.A.; van den Heuvel, B.; Bonjer, H.J.; Anema, J.R.; Huirne, J.A.F. Using E-Health in Perioperative Care: A Survey Study Investigating Shortcomings in Current Perioperative Care and Possible Future Solutions. *BMC Surg.* **2017**, *17*, 61. [CrossRef] [PubMed]

16. Timmers, T.; Janssen, L.; van der Weegen, W.; Das, D.; Marijnissen, W.-J.; Hannink, G.; van der Zwaard, B.C.; Plat, A.; Thomassen, B.; Swen, J.-W.; et al. The Effect of an App for Day-to-Day Postoperative Care Education on Patients With Total Knee Replacement: Randomized Controlled Trial. *JMIR mHealth uHealth* **2019**, *7*, e15323. [CrossRef] [PubMed]

17. Hardwick-Morris, M.; Carlton, S.; Twiggs, J.; Miles, B.; Liu, D. Pre- and Postoperative Physiotherapy Using a Digital Application Decreases Length of Stay without Reducing Patient Outcomes Following Total Knee Arthroplasty. *Arthroplasty* **2022**, *4*, 30. [CrossRef]

18. Delgado, D.A.; Lambert, B.S.; Boutris, N.; McCulloch, P.C.; Robbins, A.B.; Moreno, M.R.; Harris, J.D. Validation of Digital Visual Analog Scale Pain Scoring With a Traditional Paper-Based Visual Analog Scale in Adults. *JAAOS Glob. Res. Rev.* **2018**, *2*, e088. [CrossRef]

19. Mahajan, A.; Esper, S.A.; Cole, D.J.; Fleisher, L.A. Anesthesiologists' Role in Value-Based Perioperative Care and Healthcare Transformation. *Anesthesiology* **2021**, *134*, 526–540. [CrossRef]

20. The Royal College of Anaesthetists PERIOPERATIVE MEDICINE the PATHWAY TO BETTER SURGICAL CARE 2015. Available online: https://www.rcoa.ac.uk/sites/default/files/documents/2019-08/Perioperative%20Medicine%20-%20The%20Pathway%20to%20Better%20Care.pdf (accessed on 10 October 2023).

21. Thurnheer, S.E.; Gravestock, I.; Pichierri, G.; Steurer, J.; Burgstaller, J.M. Benefits of Mobile Apps in Pain Management: Systematic Review. *JMIR mHealth uHealth* **2018**, *6*, e11231. [CrossRef]

22. Khalid, S.; Mohammad, H.R.; Gooberman-Hill, R.; Garriga, C.; Pinedo-Villanueva, R.; Arden, N.; Price, A.; Wylde, V.; Peters, T.J.; Blom, A.; et al. Post-Operative Determinants of Chronic Pain after Primary Knee Replacement Surgery: Analysis of Data on 258,386 Patients from the National Joint Registry for England, Wales, Northern Ireland and the Isle of Man (NJR). *Osteoarthr. Cartil. Open* **2021**, *3*, 100139. [CrossRef] [PubMed]

23. Gungor, S.; Fields, K.; Aiyer, R.; Valle, A.G.D.; Su, E.P. Incidence and Risk Factors for Development of Persistent Postsurgical Pain Following Total Knee Arthroplasty: A Retrospective Cohort Study. *Medicine* **2019**, *98*, e16450. [CrossRef] [PubMed]

24. Jensen, M.P.; Chen, C.; Brugger, A.M. Interpretation of Visual Analog Scale Ratings and Change Scores: A Reanalysis of Two Clinical Trials of Postoperative Pain. *J. Pain* **2003**, *4*, 407–414. [CrossRef] [PubMed]

25. Grosu, I.; Thienpont, E.; De Kock, M.; Scholtes, J.L.; Lavand'homme, P. Dynamic View of Postoperative Pain Evolution after Total Knee Arthroplasty: A Prospective Observational Study. *Minerva Anestesiol.* **2016**, *82*, 274–283.

26. Althaus, A.; Arránz Becker, O.; Neugebauer, E. Distinguishing between Pain Intensity and Pain Resolution: Using Acute Post-Surgical Pain Trajectories to Predict Chronic Post-Surgical Pain. *Eur. J. Pain* **2014**, *18*, 513–521. [CrossRef] [PubMed]

27. Wylde, V.; Beswick, A.D.; Dennis, J.; Gooberman-Hill, R. Post-Operative Patient-Related Risk Factors for Chronic Pain after Total Knee Replacement: A Systematic Review. *BMJ Open* **2017**, *7*, e018105. [CrossRef] [PubMed]

28. van Driel, M.E.C.; van Dijk, J.F.M.; Baart, S.J.; Meissner, W.; Huygen, F.J.P.M.; Rijsdijk, M. Development and Validation of a Multivariable Prediction Model for Early Prediction of Chronic Postsurgical Pain in Adults: A Prospective Cohort Study. *Br. J. Anaesth.* **2022**, *129*, 407–415. [CrossRef]

29. Burns, L.C.; Ritvo, S.E.; Ferguson, M.K.; Clarke, H.; Seltzer, Z.; Katz, J. Pain Catastrophizing as a Risk Factor for Chronic Pain after Total Knee Arthroplasty: A Systematic Review. *J. Pain Res.* **2015**, *8*, 21–32. [CrossRef]

30. Lenguerrand, E.; Wylde, V.; Gooberman-Hill, R.; Sayers, A.; Brunton, L.; Beswick, A.D.; Dieppe, P.; Blom, A.W. Trajectories of Pain and Function after Primary Hip and Knee Arthroplasty: The ADAPT Cohort Study. *PLoS ONE* **2016**, *11*, e0149306. [CrossRef]

31. Bade, M.J.; Kohrt, W.M.; Stevens-Lapsley, J.E. Outcomes Before and After Total Knee Arthroplasty Compared to Healthy Adults. *J. Orthop. Sports Phys. Ther.* **2010**, *40*, 559–567. [CrossRef]

32. Lewis, G.N.; Rice, D.A.; Rashid, U.; McNair, P.J.; Kluger, M.T.; Somogyi, A.A. Trajectories of Pain and Function Outcomes up to 5 to 8 Years Following Total Knee Arthroplasty. *J. Arthroplast.* **2023**, *38*, 1516–1521. [CrossRef] [PubMed]

33. Sun, X.-L.; Zhao, Z.-H.; Ma, J.-X.; Li, F.-B.; Li, Y.-J.; Meng, X.-M.; Ma, X.-L. Continuous Local Infiltration Analgesia for Pain Control After Total Knee Arthroplasty: A Meta-Analysis of Randomized Controlled Trials. *Medicine* **2015**, *94*, e2005. [CrossRef] [PubMed]

34. Xing, Q.; Dai, W.; Zhao, D.; Wu, J.; Huang, C.; Zhao, Y. Adductor Canal Block with Local Infiltrative Analgesia Compared with Local Infiltrate Analgesia for Pain Control after Total Knee Arthroplasty: A Meta-Analysis of Randomized Controlled Trials. *Medicine* **2017**, *96*, e8103. [CrossRef] [PubMed]

35. Youm, Y.S.; Cho, S.D.; Cho, H.Y.; Hwang, C.H.; Jung, S.H.; Kim, K.H. Preemptive Femoral Nerve Block Could Reduce the Rebound Pain After Periarticular Injection in Total Knee Arthroplasty. *J. Arthroplast.* **2016**, *31*, 1722–1726. [CrossRef] [PubMed]

36. Levene, J.L.; Weinstein, E.J.; Cohen, M.S.; Andreae, D.A.; Chao, J.Y.; Johnson, M.; Hall, C.B.; Andreae, M.H. Local Anesthetics and Regional Anesthesia versus Conventional Analgesia for Preventing Persistent Postoperative Pain in Adults and Children: A Cochrane Systematic Review and Meta-Analysis Update. *J. Clin. Anesth.* **2019**, *55*, 116–127. [CrossRef] [PubMed]

37. Kukreja, P.; Paul, L.M.; Sellers, A.R.; Nagi, P.; Kalagara, H. The Role of Regional Anesthesia in the Development of Chronic Pain: A Review of Literature. *Curr. Anesthesiol. Rep.* **2022**, *12*, 417–438. [CrossRef]

38. Kim, H.-J.; Roychoudhury, P.; Lohia, S.; Kim, J.-S.; Kim, H.-T.; Ro, Y.-J.; Koh, W.-U. Comparison of General and Spinal Anaesthesia on Systemic Inflammatory Response in Patients Undergoing Total Knee Arthroplasty: A Propensity Score Matching Analysis. *Medicina* **2021**, *57*, 1250. [CrossRef]

39. Wickline, A.; Cole, W.; Melin, M.; Ehmann, S.; Aviles, F.; Bradt, J. Mitigating the Post-Operative Swelling Tsunami in Total Knee Arthroplasty: A Call to Action. *J Orthop. Exp. Innov.* **2023**. [CrossRef]

40. McDowell, M.; Park, A.; Gerlinger, T.L. The Painful Total Knee Arthroplasty. *Orthop. Clin. N. Am.* **2016**, *47*, 317–326. [CrossRef]

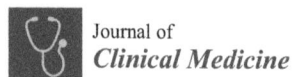

Journal of
Clinical Medicine

Article

The Role of Ketamine as a Component of Multimodal Analgesia in Burns: A Retrospective Observational Study

Marina Stojanović [1,2,†], Milana Marinković [3,*,†], Biljana Miličić [4], Milan Stojičić [1,3], Marko Jović [1,3], Milan Jovanović [1,3], Jelena Isaković Subotić [3], Milana Jurišić [3], Miodrag Karamarković [3], Aleksandra Đekić [3], Kristina Radenović [3], Jovan Mihaljević [3], Ivan Radosavljević [3], Branko Suđecki [3], Milan Savić [1,5], Marko Kostić [1,5], Željko Garabinović [1,5] and Jelena Jeremić [1,3]

1 Faculty of Medicine, University of Belgrade, 11000 Belgrade, Serbia
2 Center for Anesthesiology and Resuscitation, University Clinical Center of Serbia, 11000 Belgrade, Serbia
3 Clinic for Burns, Plastic and Reconstructive Surgery, University Clinical Center of Serbia, 11000 Belgrade, Serbia
4 Department of Medical Statistics and Informatics, School of Dental Medicine, University of Belgrade, 11000 Belgrade, Serbia
5 Clinic for Thoracic Surgery, University Clinical Center of Serbia, 11000 Belgrade, Serbia
* Correspondence: milana94pv@hotmail.com; Tel.: +381-644958190
† These authors contributed equally to this work.

Citation: Stojanović, M.; Marinković, M.; Miličić, B.; Stojičić, M.; Jović, M.; Jovanović, M.; Isaković Subotić, J.; Jurišić, M.; Karamarković, M.; Đekić, A.; et al. The Role of Ketamine as a Component of Multimodal Analgesia in Burns: A Retrospective Observational Study. *J. Clin. Med.* 2024, 13, 764. https://doi.org/10.3390/jcm13030764

Academic Editors: Patrice Forget, Felice Eugenio Agro, Giuseppe Pascarella and Fabio Costa

Received: 27 December 2023
Revised: 19 January 2024
Accepted: 23 January 2024
Published: 29 January 2024

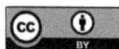
Abstract: Background: Burn wound dressing and debridement are excruciatingly painful procedures that call for appropriate analgesia—typically multimodal. Better post-procedural pain management, less opioid use, and consequently fewer side effects, which could prolong recovery and increase morbidity, are all benefits of this type of analgesia. Intravenously administered ketamine can be effective as monotherapy or in combination with opioids, especially with procedural sedation such as in burn wound dressing. **Methods**: This observational study investigated the effect of ketamine administered in subanesthetic doses combined with opioids during burn wound dressing. The study was conducted from October 2018 to October 2021. A total of 165 patients met the inclusion criteria. A total of 82 patients were in the ketamine group, while 83 patients were dressed without ketamine. The main outcome was the effect of ketamine on intraprocedural opioid consumption. The secondary outcome included the effect of ketamine on postprocedural pain control. **Results**: Patients dressed with ketamine were significantly older ($p = 0.001$), while the mean doses of intraoperatively administered propofol and fentanyl were significantly lower than in patients dressed without ketamine (150 vs. 220 mg, $p < 0.001$; and 0.075 vs. 0.150 mg, $p < 0.001$; respectively). **Conclusions**: Ketamine was an independent predictor of lower intraoperative fentanyl consumption, according to the multivariate regression analysis ($p = 0.015$). Contrarily, both groups of patients required postoperative tramadol treatment, while intraoperative ketamine administration had no beneficial effects on postoperative pain management.

Keywords: acute pain control; burns; burn wound dressing; multimodal analgesia; opioid consumption; postoperative analgesia; postoperative pain; ketamine

1. Introduction

Burns present some of the most painful injuries; thus, pain control in such trauma remains challenging and demanding [1]. The importance of effective acute burn pain management is reflected in the reduction in acute suffering as well as the prevention of neuropathic and chronic pain [2].

When selecting an analgesic, it is important to consider the changes that take place during the acute phase of a burn injury. These changes include decreased blood flow through tissues, which lowers drug clearance, changes in acute phase protein concentration, which affects drug binding to proteins, as well as metabolic changes and volume shifts [1].

The American Burn Association Guidelines (ABA) state that a variety of drugs, including opioids, non-steroidal anti-inflammatory drugs (NSAIDs), gabapentin, pregabalin, alpha-2 agonists, lidocaine, and ketamine, can be used to treat pain in burn patients [1]. Lidocaine given intravenously ought to be used as a second- or third-line adjuvant analgesic [1].

Burn wound dressing and debridement are extremely painful procedures that call for appropriate analgesia—typically multimodal. The combination of medications with various but complementary or additive mechanisms of action is suggested by the multimodal analgesia principle in order to provide the optimal pain management [3]. Better post-procedural pain management, less opioid use, and consequently fewer side effects, which could prolong recovery and increase morbidity, are all benefits of this type of analgesia [3–5]. Despite studies that demonstrate the effectiveness of multimodal analgesia in reducing postoperative pain, it is important to consider both the patient's specific pain response and the pain mechanism particular to the treatment when selecting non-opioid medications [5].

There exists a growing interest in the use of ketamine for the management of acute pain to reduce the dose-dependent adverse effects of opioids [1]. Ketamine induces dissociative anesthesia with effects of sedation, amnesia, and pain relief [6]. Intravenously administered ketamine can be effective as monotherapy or in combination with opioids, especially with procedural sedation such as in burn wound dressing, as it is a non-competitive N-methyl d-aspartate (NMDA) receptor antagonist with anesthetic, analgesic, anti-inflammatory, and antidepressant effects [7–9]. Ketamine is a drug of choice for short-term procedures when muscle relaxation is not required [10]. A patient's management of acute trauma pain might be complicated due to the patient's mental state, age, or alteration in their state of consciousness [11]. Ketamine is frequently used in severely injured patients and appears to be safe in this group. It has been widely used for emergency surgery in field conditions in war zones [12]. A 2011 clinical practice guideline supports the use of ketamine as a sedative in emergency medicine, including during physically painful procedures [13].

Another benefit of ketamine is reflected in its characteristic of not inducing hypotension or bradycardia [14,15]. Ketamine releases catecholamines by inhibiting neuronal and extraneuronal reuptake, raising cardiac output, heart rate, and arterial pressure [15]. White et al. found that during anesthesia induction ketamine increased mean arterial pressure by 10% [15]. According to clinical practice guidelines, ketamine is the drug of choice for people in traumatic shock who are at risk of hypotension [13]. It is also frequently used to provide analgesia and anesthesia to patients with hemodynamic instability and to morbidly obese patients who require high opioid doses [3,16]. Burn shock incorporates distributive, hypovolemic, and cardiogenic features, and is characterized by a diffuse capillary leak in which electrolytes, proteins, and plasma decrease the volume of the circulatory system, as well as interfere with end-organ perfusion, leading to cellular hypoxia [17–19]. Considering the circulatory changes as well as the high risk of hemodynamic instability, the use of ketamine for short-term procedures such as wound dressing in burn patients would have great benefits. Even though it has been used as an anesthetic for years, there is a lack of data showing the effect of subanesthetic doses of ketamine combined with opioids during burn wound dressing. Thus, further studies are still needed to elucidate their indications in this context.

The aims of this study are to examine the effect of ketamine administered during burn wound dressing on intraprocedural opioid consumption, particularly its effect in relation to burn size and depth, as well as its effect on postprocedural pain control.

2. Materials and Methods

2.1. Study Design and Population

This study was designed as a retrospective observational study and included patients with burn injuries treated at the Clinic for Burns, Plastic, and Reconstructive Surgery, University Clinical Centre of Serbia in Belgrade in the period from October 2018 to October 2021. The study was approved by the Institutional Review Board (date 20 September 2021, approval number 415/66) and performed in accordance with the tenets of the Declaration of Helsinki. Inclusion criteria were patients of both sexes, older than 15 years, with burn injuries of various extents, who required burn wound dressings and debridement in the operating room under intravenous anesthesia between the 3rd and the 5th day post-injury (following the initial 48 h of hemodynamic stabilization and before the planned definitive surgical treatment). Patients with superficial partial-thickness burns, deep partial-thickness burns, as well as patients with a combination of deep and superficial burns, were included. Of the 295 patients admitted to the burn unit, 165 met the inclusion criteria for the study while 130 patients were excluded from the study. Patients with inhalation injuries, intubated patients on mechanical ventilation, and patients with well-known contraindications for the use of ketamine were excluded. Due to the pathophysiological response to pain in deep burns, patients with full-thickness burns were also excluded from the study. Another exclusion criterion was insufficient postoperative pain data (Figure 1).

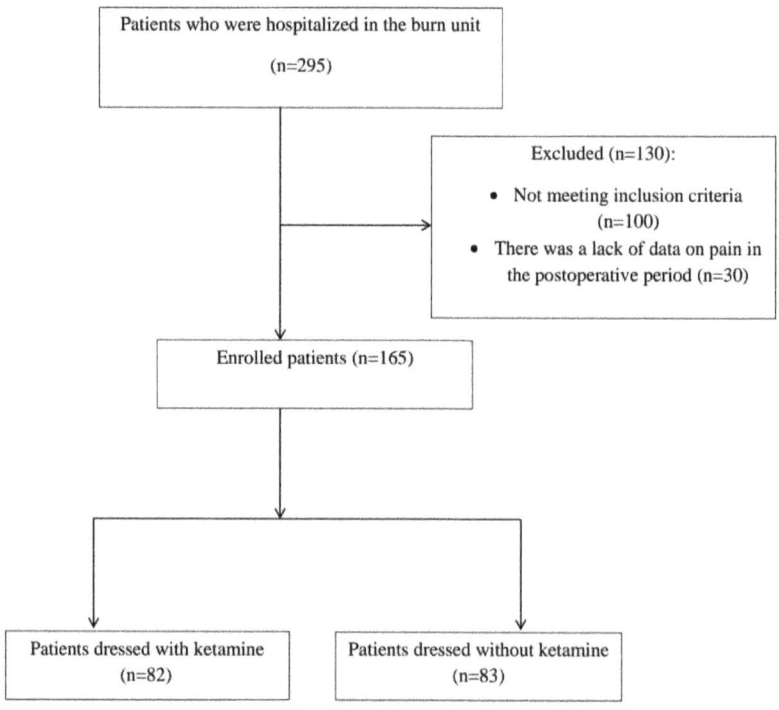

Figure 1. Flow chart of the study. A total of 130 of the 295 patients were excluded from the study. A total of 165 of patients met the inclusion criteria. A total of 82 of the included patients were dressed with ketamine, while 83 were dressed without ketamine.

2.2. Anesthetic Management

The choice of anesthetic management was decided by the senior anesthesiologists. All patients received premedication of 0.1 mg/kg midazolam and 0.5 mg atropine intramuscularly, 30 min before the burn wound dressing was performed. The position of the patient on the operating table depended on the location of the burns and included a back position, a side position, and a prone position. To secure the airway, laryngeal masks of appropriate size were used, while anesthesia was maintained with a gas mixture of air (2 L/min) and oxygen (2 L/min).

Patients were divided into two groups based on whether they received ketamine during burn dressing: 82 patients in the ketamine group and 83 patients in the non-ketamine group. A subanesthetic dose of ketamine (0.5 mg/kg) was prescribed to patients in the ketamine group at the beginning of the intervention. Patients from both groups received fentanyl and propofol in a dose individually determined by their requirements during the burn wound dressing. The depth of the burn injury, the total body surface area burned (TBSA), the age and sex of the patient, the duration of the treatment, as well as the impact of the administration of subanesthetic doses of ketamine (0.5 mg/kg) on the intraoperative requirements for opioid analgesics (fentanyl), were noted.

After burn wound dressing was performed, the patients were admitted to the intensive care unit (ICU). Standard hemodynamic parameters (pulse rate, blood pressure, oxygen saturation), and electrocardiogram (ECG) were continuously monitored and recorded every hour during the first 24 h after the procedure. Standard laboratory variables such as blood counts, coagulation status, and biochemical analyses were checked.

Pain intensity at rest was measured using the numerical pain intensity scale (NPIS) 1 h, 3 h, 6 h, 12 h, and 24 h after wound dressing. The intensity of pain in motion was not measured, considering the fact that different parts of the body were affected by burns, and it was thus not possible to define a specific motion that would be valid for all patients. A combination of NSAIDs and paracetamol was used for postprocedural analgesia; thus, all patients received paracetamol 1 g and ketorolac 30 mg every 8 h during the first 24 h. In patients whose non-opioid analgesic therapy was not satisfactory (when the intensity of pain on the NPIS scale was over 4), tramadol was prescribed in a dose of 100 mg, which was repeated according to the patient's requirements. Additionally, the impact of intraprocedurally administered ketamine on the need for additional postoperative analgesia and the need for postoperative tramadol was examined.

2.3. Study Outcomes and Data Collection

The main outcome was assessing the effect of ketamine on intraprocedural opioid consumption, while the secondary outcome included the effect of ketamine on postprocedural pain control. Demographics, medical histories, and perioperative variable data, including the type and amount of anaesthetic used, pain intensity, as well as the need for additional analgetic, were collected from medical records. Due to the lack of information, the side effects of ketamine could not be analyzed.

2.4. Statistical Analysis

SPSS software for Windows version 20.0 was used for statistical data analysis. Numerical variables are shown in the form of mean values ± standard deviation, coefficient of variation, and minimum and maximum values, while categorical variables are shown as absolute numbers and percentages. Using the Kolmogorov–Smirnov test, the normality of the data distribution was checked. Pearson's χ^2 test (contingency tables) was used to analyze data with normal distribution, while the Mann–Whitney U test was used to analyze data without normal distribution. Predictors of differences between the analyzed groups of patients (the group without ketamine and the group with ketamine) were determined by logistic regression analysis. Values of $p < 0.05$ were considered statistically significant.

3. Results

Of the 165 patients included in the study, 63% were male while 37% were female. The mean age was 51.86 ± 11.42 years (the youngest patient was 15 years old, while the oldest was 93). The mean TBSA was $23.97 \pm 15.45\%$, with the least TBSA burned being 3%, and the largest TBSA burned being 66%. According to TBSA burned, patients were divided into 6 groups (TBSA less than 10%, TBSA 11–20%, TBSA 21–30%, TBSA 31–40%, TBSA 41–50%, and TBSA above 50%). Most patients (33.9%) were in the 11–20% TBSA burned group, while the fewest (6.1%) were in the 41–50% TBSA burned group. There were about 10.3% of patients with burns greater than 50% TBSA. The patients' characteristics are shown in Table 1.

There was no statistical significance in the difference between the genders in the ketamine and the non-ketamine group. Patients in the ketamine group were significantly younger (46.03 ± 19.59 vs. 55.38 ± 17.95, $p = 0.001$, Mann–Whitney U test). However, there were no differences between groups according to TBSA burned (p = 0.733, Mann–Whitney U test).

Table 1. Patients' characteristics.

Variable	N (%)
Included patients	165 (100%)
Age (mean ± SD), years	51.86 ± 11.42
Sex: male	104 (63.0%)
TBSA burned (mean ± SD)%	23.97 ± 15.45%
Patients with TBSA burned <10%	25 (15.2%)
Patients with TBSA burned 11–20%	56 (33.9%)
Patients with TBSA burned 21–30%	39 (23.6%)
Patients with TBSA burned 31–40%	18 (10.9%)
Patients with TBSA burned 41–50%	10 (6.1%)
Patients with TBSA burned >51%	17 (10.3%)

SD—standard deviation; N—number of patients; TBSA—total body surface area.

The mean body weight in the ketamine group was 71.94 ± 8.04, while in the non-ketamine group it was 72.95 ± 7.55, with no statistical difference (p = 0.393, Mann–Whitney U test). The median dose of intraoperatively administered propofol in the ketamine group was 150 mg (minimum 0 mg, maximum 480 mg), compared to the 220 mg (minimum 70 mg, maximum 500 mg) in the non-ketamine group, with a statistically significant difference ($p < 0.01$, Mann–Whitney U test). Additionally, patients in the ketamine group received significantly lower doses of fentanyl during wound dressing than patients in the non-ketamine group (0.075 mg vs. 0.150 mg, $p < 0.01$, Mann–Whitney U test) (Table 2).

Table 2. Characteristics of patients dressed with and without ketamine.

Variable	With Ketamine N (%)	Without Ketamine N(%)	p Value
Patients	82 (49.7%)	83 (50.3%)	
Age (mean ± SD), years	46.0.3 ± 19.59	55.38 ± 17.95	0.001
Sex:			
male	52 (31.5%)	52 (31.5%)	0.599
TBSA burned (mean ± SD)%	24.75 ± 16.27	23.37 ± 14.84	0.733
TBSA% subgroups:			0.918
TBSA burned <10%	13 (7.9%)	11 (6.7%)	
TBSA burned 11–20%	26 (15.8%)	30 (18.2%)	
TBSA burned 21–30%	18 (10.9%)	21 (12.7%)	
TBSA burned 31–40%	9 (5.5%)	10 (6.1%)	
TBSA burned 41–50%	7 (4.2%)	3 (1.8%)	
TBSA burned >51%	9 (5.4%)	8 (4.8%)	
Body wight (mean ± SD), kg	71.94 ± 8.04	72.95 ± 7.55	0.393
Fentanyl median (range) mg	0.075 (0.00–0.40)	0.150 (0.05–0.50)	<0.001
Propofol, median (range) mg	150 (0–480)	220 (70–500)	<0.001
Tramadol postoperatively			0.631
Yes	30 (18.2%)	24 (14.5%)	

SD—standard deviation; N—number of patients; TBSA—total body surface area.

Although rest pain intensity measured by NPIS was lower in the first 12 h after wound dressing in the ketamine group, statistical significance was not observed compared to the non-ketamine group (Table 3). About 32.7% of patients received tramadol in the postoperative period, while 67.3% of patients did not require additional analgesia. The requirement for tramadol was quite uniform in patients who received intraoperative ketamine, compared with the patients who did not receive intraoperative ketamine (p = 0.631, Pearson χ^2 test) (Table 2).

Table 3. Rest pain intensity measured with numerical pain intensity scale 1 h, 3 h, 6 h, 12 h, and 24 h after procedure. No statistical significance was observed between two groups.

Variable	With Ketamine	Without Ketamine	*p* Value
Rest pain 1 h after procedure	1.8 ± 0.2	2.2 ± 0.2	0.691
Rest pain 3 h after procedure	3.3 ± 0.7	3.6 ± 0.2	0.851
Rest pain 6 h after procedure	5.0 ± 0.2	5.4 ± 0.6	0.776
Rest pain 12 h after procedure	5.3 ± 0.1	5.5 ± 0.3	0.966
Rest pain 24 h after procedure	3.8 ± 0.4	3.7 ± 0.3	0.899

The logistic regression analysis showed that patients who received ketamine during burn wound dressing were significantly older; moreover, they received significantly lower doses of both propofol and fentanyl than patients who did not receive ketamine (Table 4). Additionally, using multivariate logistic regression analysis, intraoperative use of ketamine was found to be an independent predictor of reduced intraoperative use of fentanyl (Table 5).

Table 4. Univariate regression analysis showed that patients who received ketamine during burn wound dressing were significantly older; moreover, they received significantly lower doses of both propofol and fentanyl than patients who did not receive ketamine.

Characteristics	OR (95% CI)	*p* Value
Gender	1.187 (0.626–2.252)	0.599
Age	1.027 (1.009–1.044)	0.002
TBSA burned	0.994 (0.975–1.014)	0.567
TBSA burned in subgruops	0.952 (0.775–1.170)	0.641
Body weight (kg)	1.017 (0.977–1.058)	0.410
Propofol (mg)	1.007 (1.003–1.010)	<0.001
Fentanyl	5247.123 (73.202–376,112.12)	<0.001

CI—confidence interval; TBSA—total body surface area.

Table 5. Multivariate regression analysis showed that intraoperative use of ketamine was an independent predictor of reduced intraoperative use of fentanyl.

Characteristics	OR (95% CI)	*p* Value
Propofol (mg)	1.005 (1.000–1.009)	0.095
Fentanyl	822.330 (3.693–183,088.334)	0.015

CI—confidence interval.

4. Discussion

This study demonstrated that when ketamine was used in subanesthetic doses (0.25–0.5 mg/kg) during burn wound dressing under intravenous anesthesia in patients with burns of various extents between the third and the fifth day after injury, the patients received lower doses of propofol and fentanyl. The study also demonstrated that ketamine was an independent predictor of decreased intraoperative fentanyl use.

In a meta-analysis, McGiness et al. demonstrated that ketamine had the best analgesic impact on burn patients when compared to other analgesics [8]. They claimed that ketamine given intravenously at a dose of 0.3 mg/kg/h considerably decreased the occurrence of secondary hyperalgesia when compared to a dose of 0.15 mg/kg/h, whereas the addition of morphine had no effect [8]. Moreover, they demonstrated that adverse effects like nausea and vomiting occurred following the injection of morphine, but sleepiness was, as anticipated, dose-dependent [8]. They did not investigate if hallucinations occurred. In this study, it was demonstrated that ketamine's coanalgesic action might be used to effectively manage pain during burn wound dressing at subanesthetic doses. However, the occurrence of side effects from ketamine were not investigated.

In patients who underwent skin grafting, Lennertz et al. investigated how perioperative multimodal analgesia affected both intraoperative and postoperative opioid consumption [20]. They demonstrated that the most significant predictors of postoperative opioid usage were age and TBSA burned [20]. Younger patients in their study required larger morphine doses; morphine intake fell by 2.7 morphine equivalents (ME) for every year of age (1 ME = 1 mg of oral morphine) [20]. They also demonstrated that for every 10% rise in TBSA burned, there was a 1.8 ME increase in opioid intake, with the average amount of opioid use rising from 166 ± 94 ME preoperatively to roughly 218 ± 117 ME in the first 24 h postoperatively [20]. Similar to our findings, this study demonstrated that the single administration of ketamine, whether as preemptive analgesia or intraoperatively, had no impact on the postoperative reduction in opioid consumption. Patients with a larger %TBSA burned are likely to require longer time in the OR necessary for burn wound dressing, resulting in a higher consumption of fentanyl which decreases the level of pain in the early post-procedural course. In this study, however, the patients who received ketamine during wound dressing had significantly lower fentanyl use; thus, a higher level of pain in the post-procedural course would be expected. Given how this study found no difference in pain intensity after dressing between the groups, it can be assumed that ketamine had some effect on pain intensity. The injection of ketamine in a bolus dose without further continuous infusion administration may be one explanation for this. The average percent of body surface area burned was higher (8.1% vs. 23.7% TBSA), and a positive correlation was found between the %TBSA burned and the intraoperative use of opioids. This was to be expected given that patients with extensive burns required more intraoperative analgesic administration due to the longer duration of burn wound dressing and the intensity of their pain.

Ketamine was utilized by Brennan et al. in a bolus dose of 1.2 mg/kg, repeated as needed for 5 min during burn wound dressing, along with benzodiazepines at an average dose of 3 mg, and opioids (fentanyl at an average dose of 10 ME) in 26% of patients [21]. Dysphoric reactions were seen in 6% of individuals, whereas the remaining 6% experienced ketamine-induced hypertension that responded positively to labetalol given intravenously [11]. They used a higher dose of ketamine (0.25–0.5 mg/kg vs. 1.2 mg/kg) and did not utilize propofol, which increased the risk of complications such as ketamine-induced hypertension [21]. In order to achieve the desired level of analgosedation during wound dressing in burn patients, Gündüz et al. investigated the effects of various drug combinations (1 mg/kg ketamine followed by 1 mg/kg dexmedetomidine, 0.05 mg/kg midazolam, and saline solution) [22]. The dexmedetomidine–ketamine combination performed better than other combinations in terms of blood pressure and heart rate, as well as analgesia and postoperative sedation duration [22]. In addition, Zor et al. analyzed the ideal analgesic combination for the dressing of burn wounds [23]. The participants in their study were split into three groups: the first received a dose of 2 mg/kg of ketamine alone; the second, 1 mg/kg of tramadol and, after 30 min, 1 g/kg of dexmedetomidine and 2 mg/kg of ketamine; and the third, 1 mg/kg of tramadol and, after 30 min, 0.05 mg/kg of midazolam and 2 mg/kg of ketamine [23]. With regard to pain management and side effects, the second group performed better [23].

Ketamine can be taken orally, rectally, or intranasally in addition to intravenously. There have been some investigations into ketamine taken orally [24,25]. Kundra et al. investigated the effects of oral ketamine (5 mg/kg) and dexmedetomidine (4 g/kg) on pain management during burn wound dressing [24]. They showed noticeably lower pain scores, with 67% in the ketamine group and 44% in the dexmedetomidine group (the mean for the groups being 2.6 ± 0.6 and 3.8 ± 0.8, respectively) [24]. In a retrospective study, Lintner et al. found that patients who received oral ketamine in doses of 0.5–3 mg/kg with 2–4 mg of midazolam as premedication had statistically significantly lower doses of intravenously administered opioids (fentanyl or hydromorphine, 50 mg vs. 75 mg, $p = 0.009$) [25]. Ketamine, whether administered orally or intravenously, reduces the requirement for intraoperative opioid consumption and, as a result, the likelihood of side effects associated with the use of opioids in large doses. Furthermore, according to Grossmann et al., children with burns less than 6% TBSA burned can achieve a satisfactory level of analgosedation with a reasonable recovery period and few side effects when receiving rectally administered ketamine at a dose of 6 mg/kg combined with 0.5 mg/kg of dormicum [26].

The effectiveness of ketamine as a coanalgesic in postoperative pain control following various types of surgery, as well as the prevalence of side effects, were evaluated by Subramaniam et al. in a meta-analysis and systematic review [27]. A total of 20 out of the 37 studies included in the analysis revealed that the addition of ketamine to opioids had a positive impact on postoperative pain management, particularly when it was given as a bolus or continuous infusion [27]. It was not demonstrated, however, how the timing of ketamine administration affected its analgesic impact (before incision, during operation, or after surgery). In individuals who had developed an acute tolerance to opioids, the favorable effects of ketamine on the lowering of pain intensity and the opioid sparing effect are described in the literature [28]. The use of ketamine was considered when the severity of postoperative pain necessitated high doses of opioids, such as in major abdominal and thoracic surgery, given how a combination of local anesthetics, NSAIDs, and opioids typically provided adequate analgesia in surgical procedures like appendectomy, tonsillectomy, laparoscopic surgery, and knee arthroscopy [27]. Additionally, the administration of ketamine had no impact on the incidence of psychomimetic side effects or the reduction in respiratory depression, pruritus, or postoperative nausea and vomiting [27].

According to Brinck et al., preoperative ketamine injection considerably decreased the need for postoperative opioids by 8 ME in the first 24 h and by 13 ME in the next 48 h [29]. Additionally, pain intensity at rest decreased by 19% during the first 24 h and by 22% during the next 48 h, whereas pain intensity during movement decreased by 14% during the initial 24 h and by 16% during the subsequent 48 h [29]. In addition, administering ketamine added a 54 min delay before the administration of the first analgesic in the postoperative phase [29]. Similar outcomes were obtained by Laskowski et al., and Wang et al., but none of them demonstrated a connection between the ketamine dose delivered and the desired outcome [30,31].

This study is limited by its retrospective nature, the single-center design, as well as a small number of participants. Additionally, the study's limitations stem from the fact that just one parameter of postprocedural rest pain was examined, which fails to take into account the multidimensional characteristics of pain pathways as well as patient-specific perceptions of pain. The use of subanesthetic doses of ketamine as part of multimodal analgesia in other, less painful procedures could produce different results in terms of even better pain control and lower postoperative pain score values, since burns are considered an extremely painful trauma and burn wound dressing and debridement are a typically very painful procedure. Furthermore, the post-procedural side effects of ketamine were not investigated in this study.

5. Conclusions

Administering ketamine intraoperatively in subanesthetic (analgesic) doses showed a considerably decreased need for intraoperative opioids. Patients with burns less than 20% TBSA burned as well as patients with burns larger than 21% TBSA burned both showed positive effects in terms of the reduction in use of opioids (fentanyl) and propofol. Ketamine was an independent predictor of lower intraoperative fentanyl use, according to the multivariate regression analysis. Contrarily, both groups of patients required postoperative tramadol treatment, while intraoperative ketamine administration had no statistically significant effects on postoperative pain management.

Author Contributions: Conceptualization, M.S. (Marina Stojanović), M.M.; methodology, M.S. (Marina Stojanović), M.M., M.S. (Milan Stojičić), M.J. (Marko Jović), M.J. (Milan Jovanović), J.J.; software, B.M.; validation, M.S. (Marina Stojanović), B.M., M.S. (Milan Stojičić), M.J. (Marko Jović), M.J. (Milan Jovanović), J.J., M.S. (Milan Savić), M.K. (Marko Kostić), Ž.G.; formal analysis, M.S. (Marina Stojanović), M.M., J.I.S., M.J. (Milana Jurišić), M.K. (Miodrag Karamarković), A.Đ., K.R., I.R., J.M., B.S.;

investigation, M.S. (Marina Stojanović), M.M., M.S. (Milan Savić), M.K. (Marko Kostić), Ž.G.; data curation, M.S. (Marina Stojanović), M.M., J.I.S., M.J. (Milana Jurišić), M.K. (Miodrag Karamarković), A.Đ., K.R., I.R., J.M., B.S.; writing—original draft preparation, M.S. (Marina Stojanović), M.M., B.M., M.J. (Milana Jurišić), A.Đ., K.R.; visualization, M.K. (Miodrag Karamarković), I.R., J.M., B.S.; supervision, J.J.; project administration, M.S. (Marina Stojanović), J.J. All authors have read and agreed to the published version of the manuscript.

Funding: This research received no external funding.

Institutional Review Board Statement: The study was conducted in accordance with the Declaration of Helsinki, and approved by the Institutional Review Board (approval number 415/66) (date 20 September 2021).

Informed Consent Statement: Not applicable.

Data Availability Statement: The data presented in this study are available on request from the corresponding author. The data are not publicly available due to Institutional research permit.

Conflicts of Interest: The authors declare no conflicts of interest.

References

1. Schwenk, E.S.; Viscusi, E.R.; Buvanendran, A.; Hurley, R.W.; Wasan, A.D.; Narouze, S.; Bhatia, A.; Davis, F.N.; Hooten, W.M.; Cohen, S.P. Consensus Guidelines on the Use of Intravenous Ketamine Infusions for Acute Pain Management from the American Society of Regional Anesthesia and Pain Medicine, the American Academy of Pain Medicine, and the American Society of Anesthesiologists. *Reg. Anesth. Pain Med.* **2018**, *43*, 1. [CrossRef] [PubMed]
2. Lang, T.C.; Zhao, R.; Kim, A.; Wijewardena, A.; Vandervord, J.; Xue, M.; Jackson, C.J. A Critical Update of the Assessment and Acute Management of Patients with Severe Burns. *Adv. Wound Care* **2019**, *8*, 607–633. [CrossRef] [PubMed]
3. Beverly, A.; Kaye, A.D.; Ljungqvist, O.; Urman, R.D. Essential Elements of Multimodal Analgesia in Enhanced Recovery after Surgery (ERAS) Guidelines. *Anesthesiol. Clin.* **2017**, *35*, e115–e143. [CrossRef] [PubMed]
4. da Silva, F.G.; Podestá, M.H.M.C.; Silva, T.C.; de Barros, C.M.; de Carvalho, B.F.V.; Dos Reis, T.M.; Espósito, M.C.; Marrafon, D.A.F.d.O.; Nogueira, D.A.; Diwan, S.; et al. Oral Pregabalin Is Effective as Preemptive Analgesia in Abdominal Hysterectomy-A Randomized Controlled Trial. *Clin. Exp. Pharmacol. Physiol.* **2023**, *50*, 256–263. [CrossRef] [PubMed]
5. Kehlet, H. Postoperative Pain, Analgesia, and Recovery-Bedfellows That Cannot Be Ignored. *Pain* **2018**, *159* (Suppl. S1), S11–S16. [CrossRef] [PubMed]
6. Biliškov, A.; Ivančev, B.; Pogorelić, Z. Effects on Recovery of Pediatric Patients Undergoing Total Intravenous Anesthesia with Propofol versus Ketofol for Short—Lasting Laparoscopic Procedures. *Children* **2021**, *8*, 610. [CrossRef]
7. MacPherson, R.D.; Woods, D.; Penfold, J. Ketamine and Midazolam Delivered by Patient-Controlled Analgesia in Relieving Pain Associated with Burns Dressings. *Clin. J. Pain* **2008**, *24*, 568–571. [CrossRef]
8. McGuinness, S.K.; Wasiak, J.; Cleland, H.; Symons, J.; Hogan, L.; Hucker, T.; Mahar, P.D. A Systematic Review of Ketamine as an Analgesic Agent in Adult Burn Injuries. *Pain Med.* **2011**, *12*, 1551–1558. [CrossRef]
9. Zanos, P.; Moaddel, R.; Morris, P.J.; Riggs, L.M.; Highland, J.N.; Georgiou, P.; Pereira, E.F.R.; Albuquerque, E.X.; Thomas, C.J.; Zarate, C.A., Jr.; et al. Ketamine and Ketamine Metabolite Pharmacology: Insights into Therapeutic Mechanisms. *Pharmacol. Rev.* **2018**, *70*, 621–660. [CrossRef]
10. Krupitsky, E. Attenuation of Ketamine Effects by Nimodipine Pretreatment in Recovering Ethanol Dependent Men Psychopharmacologic Implications of the Interaction of NMDA and L-Type Calcium Channel Antagonists. *Neuropsychopharmacology* **2001**, *25*, 936–947. [CrossRef]
11. Fabbri, A.; Voza, A.; Riccardi, A.; Serra, S.; Iaco, F. The Pain Management of Trauma Patients in the Emergency Department. *J. Clin. Med.* **2023**, *12*, 3289. [CrossRef]
12. Cohen, L.; Athaide, V.; Wickham, M.E.; Doyle-Waters, M.M.; Rose, N.G.W.; Hohl, C.M. The Effect of Ketamine on Intracranial and Cerebral Perfusion Pressure and Health Outcomes: A Systematic Review. *Ann. Emerg. Med.* **2015**, *65*, 43–51.e2. [CrossRef]
13. Green, S.M.; Roback, M.G.; Kennedy, R.M.; Krauss, B. Clinical Practice Guideline for Emergency Department Ketamine Dissociative Sedation: 2011 Update. *Ann. Emerg. Med.* **2011**, *57*, 449–461. [CrossRef] [PubMed]
14. White, P.F. Comparative Evaluation of Intravenous Agents for Rapid Sequence Induction—Thiopental, Ketamine, and Midazolam. *Anesthesiology* **1982**, *57*, 279–284. [CrossRef] [PubMed]
15. Ishimaru, T.; Goto, T.; Takahashi, J.; Okamoto, H.; Hagiwara, Y.; Watase, H.; Hasegawa, K.; Morita, H.; Kawano, T.; Kamikawa, Y.; et al. Author Correction: Association of Ketamine Use with Lower Risks of Post-Intubation Hypotension in Hemodynamically-Unstable Patients in the Emergency Department. *Sci. Rep.* **2020**, *10*, 2208. [CrossRef]
16. Chaouch, M.A.M.A.; Daghmouri, M.A.; Boutron, M.-C.; Ferraz, J.-M.; Usai, S.; Soubrane, O.; Beaussier, M.; Pourcher, G.; Oweira, H. Ketamine as a Component of Multimodal Analgesia for Pain Management in Bariatric Surgery: A Systematic Review and Meta-Analysis of Randomized Controlled Trials. *Ann. Med. Surg.* **2022**, *78*, 103783. [CrossRef] [PubMed]

17. Jeschke, M.G.; van Baar, M.E.; Choudhry, M.A.; Chung, K.K.; Gibran, N.S.; Logsetty, S. Burn Injury. *Nat. Rev. Dis. Primers* **2020**, *6*, 11. [CrossRef] [PubMed]
18. Rae, L.; Fidler, P.; Gibran, N. The Physiologic Basis of Burn Shock and the Need for Aggressive Fluid Resuscitation. *Crit. Care Clin.* **2016**, *32*, 491–505. [CrossRef]
19. Guillory, A.; Clayton, R.; Herndon, D.; Finnerty, C. Cardiovascular Dysfunction Following Burn Injury: What We Have Learned from Rat and Mouse Models. *Int. J. Mol. Sci.* **2016**, *17*, 53. [CrossRef]
20. Lennertz, R.; Zimmerman, H.; McCormick, T.; Hetzel, S.; Faucher, L.; Gibson, A. Perioperative Multimodal Analgesia Reduces Opioid Use Following Skin Grafting in Nonintubated Burn Patients. *J. Burn. Care Res.* **2020**, *41*, 1202–1206. [CrossRef]
21. Phg, B.; Landry, J.K.; Miles, V.P. Intravenous Ketamine as an Adjunct to Procedural Sedation during Burn Wound Care and Dressing Changes. *J. Burn Care Res.* **2019**, *40*, 246–250.
22. Gündüz, M.; Sakalli, S.; Güneş, Y.; Kesiktaş, E.; Ozcengiz, D.; Işik, G. Comparison of Effects of Ketamine, Ketamine-Dexmedetomidine and Ketamine-Midazolam on Dressing Changes of Burn Patients. *J. Anaesthesiol. Clin. Pharmacol.* **2011**, *27*, 220–224. [CrossRef]
23. Zora, F.; Ozturka, S.; Bilginb, F. Pain Relief during Dressing Changes of Major Adult Burns: Ideal Analgesic Combination with Ketamine. *Burns* **2010**, *36*, 501–505. [CrossRef] [PubMed]
24. Kundra, P.; Velayudhana, S.; Krishnamacharib, S. Oral Ketamine and Dexmedetomidine in Adults' Burns Wound Dressing-A Randomized Double Blind Cross over Study. *Burns* **2013**, *39*, 1150–1156. [CrossRef] [PubMed]
25. Lintner, A.C.; Brennan, P.; Miles, M.V.P.; Leonard, C.; Alexander, K.M.; Kahn, S.A. Oral Administration of Injectable Ketamine during Burn Wound Dressing Changes. *J. Pharm. Pract.* **2021**, *34*, 423–427. [CrossRef] [PubMed]
26. Grossmann, B.; Nilsson, A.; Sjöberg, F.; Nilsson, L. Rectal Ketamine during Paediatric Burn Wound Dressing Procedures: A Randomised Dose-Finding Study. *Burns* **2019**, *45*, 1081–1088. [CrossRef]
27. Subramaniam, K.; Subramaniam, B.; Steinbrook, R.A. Ketamine as Adjuvant Analgesic to Opioids: A Quantitative and Qualitative Systematic Review. *Anesth. Analg.* **2004**, *99*, 482–495. [CrossRef]
28. Weinbroum, A.A. A Single Small Dose of Postoperative Ketamine Provides Rapid and Sustained Improvement in Morphine Analgesia in the Presence of Morphine-Resistant Pain. *Anesth. Analg.* **2003**, *96*, 789–795. [CrossRef] [PubMed]
29. Brinck, E.C.; Tiippana, E.; Heesen, M.; Bell, R.F.; Straube, S.; Moore, R.A.; Kontinen, V. Perioperative Intravenous Ketamine for Acute Postoperative Pain in Adults. *Cochrane Database Syst. Rev.* **2018**, *12*, CD012033. [CrossRef]
30. Laskowski, K.; Stirling, A.; McKay, W.P.; Lim, H.J. A Systematic Review of Intravenous Ketamine for Postoperative Analgesia. *Can. J. Anaesth.* **2011**, *58*, 911–923. [CrossRef]
31. Wang, X.; Lin, C.; Lan, L.; Liu, J. Perioperative Intravenous S-Ketamine for Acute Postoperative Pain in Adults: A Systematic Review and Meta-Analysis. *J. Clin. Anesth.* **2021**, *68*, 110071. [CrossRef] [PubMed]

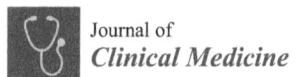

Journal of
Clinical Medicine

MDPI

Article

Lateral Femoral Cutaneous Nerve Block or Wound Infiltration Combined with Pericapsular Nerve Group (PENG) Block for Postoperative Analgesia following Total Hip Arthroplasty through Posterior Approach: A Randomized Controlled Trial

Giuseppe Pascarella [1], Fabio Costa [1], Alessandro Strumia [1,*], Alessandro Ruggiero [2], Luigi Maria Remore [1], Tullio Lanteri [1], Anton Hazboun [1], Ferdinando Longo [1], Francesca Gargano [1], Lorenzo Schiavoni [1], Alessia Mattei [1], Felice Eugenio Agrò [1,2], Massimiliano Carassiti [1,2] and Rita Cataldo [1,2]

1   Unit of Anesthesia and Intensive Care, Fondazione Policlinico Universitario Campus Bio-Medico, 00128 Rome, Italy; g.pascarella@policlinicocampus.it (G.P.); f.costa@policlinicocampus.it (F.C.); l.remore@policlinicocampus.it (L.M.R.); t.lanteri@policlinicocampus.it (T.L.); a.hazboun@policlinicocampus.it (A.H.); f.longo@policlinicocampus.it (F.L.); f.gargano@policlinicocampus.it (F.G.); l.schiavoni@policlinicocampus.it (L.S.); a.mattei@policlinicocampus.it (A.M.); f.agro@policlinicocampus.it (F.E.A.); m.carassiti@policlinicocampus.it (M.C.); r.cataldo@policlinicocampus.it (R.C.)
2   Unit of Anesthesia and Intensive Care, Department of Medicine, Università Campus Bio-Medico, 00128 Rome, Italy; alessandro.ruggiero@unicampus.it
*   Correspondence: a.strumia@policlinicocampus.it; Tel.: +39-34-7140-3574

Abstract: Background: Pericapsular nerve group (PENG) block, although effective for pain management following total hip arthroplasty (THA), does not cover skin analgesia. In this randomized controlled trial, we compared the effectiveness of PENG block combined with lateral femoral cutaneous nerve (LFCN) block or wound infiltration (WI) on postoperative analgesia and functional outcomes. **Methods:** Fifty patients undergoing posterior-approached THA under spinal anesthesia were randomly allocated to receive LFCN block with 10 mL of 0.5% ropivacaine or WI with 20 mL of 0.5% ropivacaine. In both groups, PENG block was performed by injecting 20 mL of 0.5% ropivacaine. Primary outcomes were static and dynamic pain scores (0–10 numeric rating scale) measured in the first 24 h after surgery. Secondary outcomes included postoperative opioid consumption, functional assessment and length of hospital stay. **Results:** Postoperative static NRS of patients receiving LFCN was higher than that of patients receiving WI at 6 h but lower at 24 h, with a median (IQR) of 3 (2–4) vs. 2 (1–2) ($p < 0.001$) and 2 (2–3) vs. 3 (3–4) ($p = 0.02$), respectively. Static pain scores at 12 h did not show significant differences, with an NRS of 3 (2–4) for WI vs. 3 (3–4) for LFCN ($p = 0.94$). Dynamic pain and range of movement followed a similar trend. No significant differences were detected in other outcomes. **Conclusions:** LFCN block was not inferior to WI for postoperative analgesia and functional recovery in association with PENG block during the first postoperative day, although it had worse short-term pain scores. Based on these results, it is reasonable to consider LFCN block as a valid alternative to WI or even a complementary technique added to WI to enhance skin analgesia during the first 24 h after THA. Future studies are expected to confirm this hypothesis and find the best combination between PENG block and other techniques to enhance analgesia after THA.

Keywords: total hip arthroplasty; analgesia; anesthesia; regional anesthesia; nerve block; postoperative pain

Citation: Pascarella, G.; Costa, F.; Strumia, A.; Ruggiero, A.; Remore, L.M.; Lanteri, T.; Hazboun, A.; Longo, F.; Gargano, F.; Schiavoni, L.; et al. Lateral Femoral Cutaneous Nerve Block or Wound Infiltration Combined with Pericapsular Nerve Group (PENG) Block for Postoperative Analgesia following Total Hip Arthroplasty through Posterior Approach: A Randomized Controlled Trial. *J. Clin. Med.* **2024**, *13*, 2674. https://doi.org/10.3390/jcm13092674

Academic Editor: Sorin J. Brull

Received: 26 March 2024
Revised: 28 April 2024
Accepted: 30 April 2024
Published: 2 May 2024

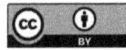
1. Introduction

Pericapsular nerve group (PENG) block is a fascial block first described in 2018 by Girón Arango and colleagues to treat hip fracture-related pain [1]. It targets periarticular sensory branches derived from the femoral, obturator and accessory obturator nerves innervating the anterior hip capsule [2]. Since 2021, many trials have been published demonstrating its efficacy in managing perioperative pain after hip arthroplasty without affecting functional recovery [3]. However, PENG block does not involve other anatomical structures affected by postsurgical stress, such as skin, periarticular fascias, muscles and posterior capsula. In particular, among all of these structures, skin has been demonstrated to have a higher concentration of nociceptors involved in hip replacement-related pain [4].

Lateral femoral cutaneous nerve (LFCN) block has been shown to contribute to cutaneous anesthesia of hip surgery incisions, although not completely [5,6]. However, these were the results of studies performed on healthy volunteers and do not take count of tissues response to surgical stress, including local inflammatory reactions which could involve tissues near the wound, although not included in the surgical incision line. Not by chance, the positive impact of LFCN block on postoperative analgesia after postero-lateral-approached THA has been confirmed by clinical investigations [7,8].

Although some authors suggest the use of LFCN combined with PENG to enhance postoperative analgesia after THA [9,10], the impact of this association has not yet been sufficiently investigated. At the same time, wound infiltration (WI) has been demonstrated to be effective in managing postoperative analgesia in different kinds of surgeries, including hip surgery [11–13].

For these reasons, we conducted a randomized controlled trial to compare the efficacy of PENG block combined with LFCN block or WI, which is our current standard treatment to cover skin analgesia following posterior THA.

2. Methods

2.1. Enrollment

This study was approved by the Ethics Committee of Campus Bio-Medico University Hospital in Rome (protocol number 34.22, date of approval: 24 May 2022) and registered on ClinicalTrials.gov (NCT05432011, Principal Investigator: Giuseppe Pascarella, Date of registration: 20 June 2022) before the first patient was enrolled. Enrollment was performed from 1 July 2022 to 18 May 2023, offered preoperatively to adults undergoing primary hip arthroplasty at the Day Surgery Department of Fondazione Policlinico Universitario Campus Bio-Medico, Italy, aged $\geq$ 18 y and ASA physical status 1–3. Patients with allergies to local anesthetics, infection of the puncture site, lack of signing of informed consent, weight < 30 kg, age < 18 years old, ASA physical status IV, dementia or cognitive impairment were excluded from this study. Fifty eligible patients were randomly allocated into two groups to receive a PENG block combined with an LFCN block or WI (Figure 1).

Randomization was achieved using computer-generated lists in blocks of eight with a 1:1 ratio, and treatment allocation was concealed using consecutively numbered, sealed, opaque envelopes. All patients underwent total hip replacement performed in the morning by the same surgical team using a posterior approach. Every patient was informed of the sequence of procedures during anesthesia and surgery, and written informed consent was obtained before enrollment.

Moreover, as part of a preoperative checklist, we always asked patients to describe both the anesthetic and surgical procedure they are undergoing in order to verify their comprehension.

In both groups, patients received mild sedation with 0.03 mg.kg^{-1} intravenous midazolam. Before surgery, 1 g acetaminophen, 30 mg ketorolac and 8 mg dexamethasone were given intravenously (i.v.) as multimodal pre-emptive analgesia. Spinal anesthesia was chosen as the main anesthetic technique. It was performed by injecting 16 mg of ropivacaine 0.5% through a 27G Whitacre needle at the L2–L3 or L3–L4 interspace with the patient in a sitting position and with the help of preprocedural ultrasound spinal evaluation [14,15].

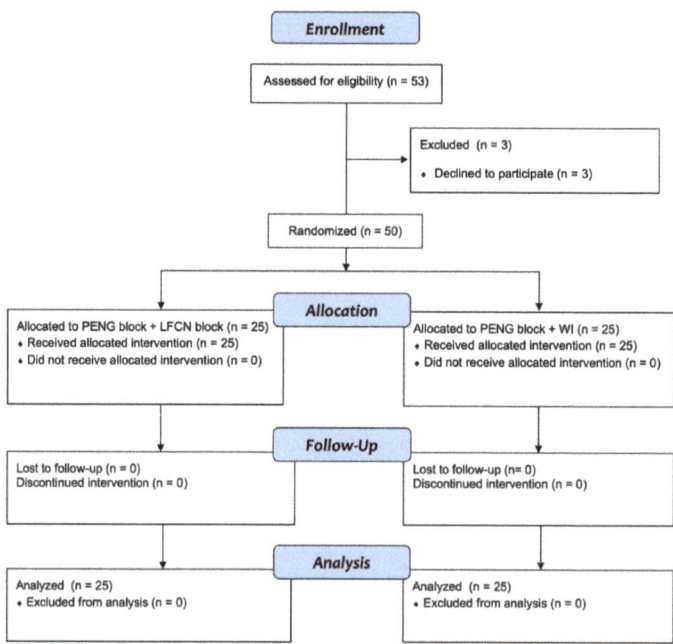

Figure 1. CONSORT flow diagram. CONSORT indicates Consolidated Standards of Reporting Trials.

2.2. Interventions

Patients were scheduled to receive WI or LFCN at the end of surgery.

WI was performed by the surgeon, injecting 20 mL of 0.5% ropivacaine in the subcutaneous tissue. Ultrasound-guided LFCN block was performed in the post-anesthesia recovery room (PACU). A linear probe was used to identify the LFCN lying between the sartorius muscle and tensor fasciae latae muscle, and then the needle (50 mm Stimuplex Ultra 360, BBraun, Melsungen, Germany) was inserted from lateral to medial to target the nerve. After a negative aspiration test, 10 mL of 0.5% ropivacaine was injected perineurally (Figure 2A). LFCN block success was assessed using an ice test on the lateral aspect of thigh at dismission from PACU.

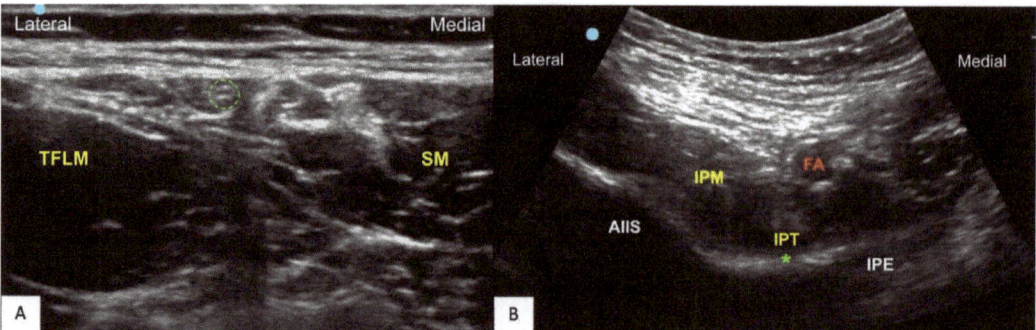

Figure 2. Regional Anesthesia Techniques: (A) Lateral femoral cutaneous nerve (LFCN) block.
Green dashed line: LFCN; TFLM: tensor fasciae latae muscle; SM: sartorius muscle **(B) PENG Block:**
IPT: iliopsoas tendon; IPE: iliopubic eminence; asterisk (green *): injection target; FA: femoral artery;
IPM: iliopsoas muscle; AIIS: anterior inferior iliac spine.

Moreover, all patients received PENG block in the PACU block according to the technique originally described by Girón-Arango [1]. A curvilinear probe was used. The needle (80 mm Stimuplex Ultra 360, BBraun, Melsungen, Germany) was inserted lateromedially until it reached the space between the iliopsoas tendon and periosteum, situated on the lateral side of the iliopubic eminence (IPE) (Figure 2B). Following confirmation via a negative aspiration test, 20 mL of 0.5% ropivacaine was injected in the plane beneath the iliopsoas muscle (IPM) to obtain transverse spread under the muscular plane with the tendon lifted [16].

PENG block and LFCN block were always performed by the same four anesthetists, (GP, FC, TL, AH) experts in regional anesthesia.

2.3. Postoperative Management

Both groups received the same postoperative multimodal analgesia, which included acetaminophen 1 g i.v. every 6 h and ketorolac 60 mg i.v. every 24 h, as recommended by international guidelines [17]. In addition, patient-controlled analgesia was provided i.v. (morphine bolus = 1 mg; lockout interval = 8 min).

2.4. Outcomes Assessment

At 6, 12 and 24 postoperative hours, patients were asked to indicate perceived static (at rest) and dynamic (hip adduction) pain using a 0–10 NRS (0 no pain, 10 worst imaginable pain).

Functional recovery of the hip joint was evaluated through the postoperative range of movement (ROM) together with the ability to perform physiotherapy and ambulation. The ROM was analyzed through active hip flexion, within the range of $0°$ to $90°$, measured with a protractor, at 6, 12, and 24 h postoperatively.

For each time point, quadriceps strength was evaluated by asking the patient to extend the leg to exclude motor paralysis due to PENG block. Furthermore, the ability to start physiotherapy and ambulate thanks to the help of a walker during the first postoperative day was recorded. In case of inability, it was specified if it was related to motor block or pain. The length of hospital stay was also recorded. We recorded any complications or side effects, including local infection, vascular puncture, nausea and/or vomiting, dizziness and respiratory depression. Outcome assessment was performed by the same group of clinicians (AS, LR, AR), blinded to patients' group allocation.

2.5. Statistical Analysis

To calculate the sample size, we focused on the primary hypothesis that postoperative analgesia after PENG block combined with LFCN is not inferior to PENG block with WI. Despite the absence of similar clinical trials at the time of our protocol study, we estimated the density of pain scores (mean 2; SD 1) based on the database of our previously published work regarding the use of PENG block combined with WI for THA [18].

To simulate power, we employed the truncated Gaussian distribution spanning from 0 to 10, with a standard deviation of 1, and a mean of 2 for the PENG + WI group. Based on these parameters and assuming a two-sided significance level of 5%, we conducted 10,000 simulations, each with a sample size of 25 per group. With a total sample size of 50 subjects, we possess 90% power to identify group disparities in pain as minimal as approximately 1. Statistical analysis and visual presentation were obtained using GraphPad Prism 8 software (GraphPad Software Inc., La Jolla, CA, USA).

Continuous quantitative variables are presented as Mean $\pm$ Standard Deviation (SD), while discrete variables are expressed as the median and interquartile range (IQR). Qualitative variables are represented by the number of observations and the percentage distribution. The parametric distribution of numerical variables was assessed using the Shapiro–Wilk normality test. Group differences for continuous parametric variables were evaluated using Student's t-test, while the Wilcoxon–Mann–Whitney U test was employed when appropriate. To mitigate the risk of type 1 error in multiple repeated measures,

Bonferroni–Dunn correction was applied. Categorical variables were compared using Pearson's chi-squared test. Statistical significance was defined as a p-value < 0.05.

3. Results

A total of 50 patients were included in the study and equally allocated between groups (Figure 2).

No clinically relevant differences were noticed between group characteristics (Table 1).

Table 1. Patient characteristics.

	PENG + LFCN (n = 25)	PENG + WI (n = 25)
Age (yrs)	67.7 ± 8.8	65.2 ± 13
Sex (M/F)	12/13	14/11
BMI (kg/m^2)	27.9 ± 3.7	28.5 ± 5.3
ASA score, n (%)		
- I	1 (4%)	2 (8%)
- II	13 (52%)	16 (64%)
- III	11 (44%)	8 (32%)
Chronic Opiate Use, n (%)		
- Yes	3 (12%)	4 (16%)
- No	22 (88%)	21 (84%)
Surgery Duration (min)	107 ± 20	105 ± 18

Values are reported as number (percentage) of subjects and mean ± standard deviation (SD). PENG: pericapsular nerve group block; LFCN: lateral femoral cutaneous nerve block; WI: wound infiltration; BMI: body mass index.

The postoperative static NRS of patients receiving LFCN was higher than that of patients receiving WI at 6 h but lower at 24 h, with a median (IQR) of 3 (2–4) vs. 2 (1–2) (p< 0.001) and 2 (2–3) vs. 3 (3–4) (p = 0.02), respectively (Figure 3).

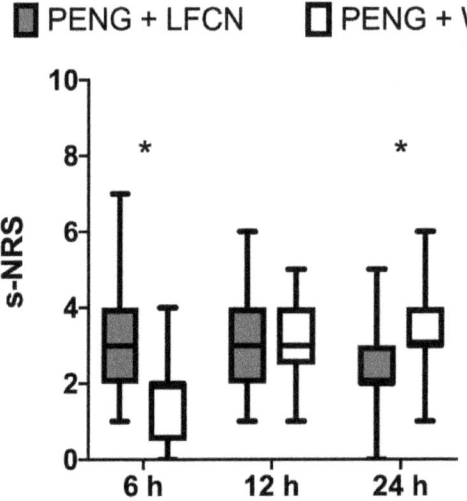

Figure 3. Static postoperative pain. The box plot shows postoperative pain scores in both study groups. Data include static pain reported at three different postoperative time points (6, 12 and 24 h).

Pain severity is expressed using a 0–10 numeric rating scale, with 0 equal to no pain and 10 being the worst imaginable pain. Values are expressed as median (horizontal bars) with 25th–75th (box) and range of minimum to maximum value (whiskers); * denotes statistical significance ($p < 0.05$). PENG: pericapsular nerve group block; WI: wound infiltration; LFCN: lateral femoral cutaneous nerve block; s-NRS: numeric rating scale at rest (static).

Static pain scores at 12 h did not show significant differences, with an NRS of 3 (2–4) for WI vs. 3 (3–4) for LFCN ($p = 0.94$). Dynamic pain scores followed a similar trend, showing a median NRS of 5 (3–6) vs. 3 (2–4) ($p < 0.001$), 4 (3–5) vs. 4 (4–5) ($p = 0.18$) and 4 (3–4) vs. 5 (4–5) ($p = 0.019$) at 6, 12, and 24 h, respectively (Figure 4).

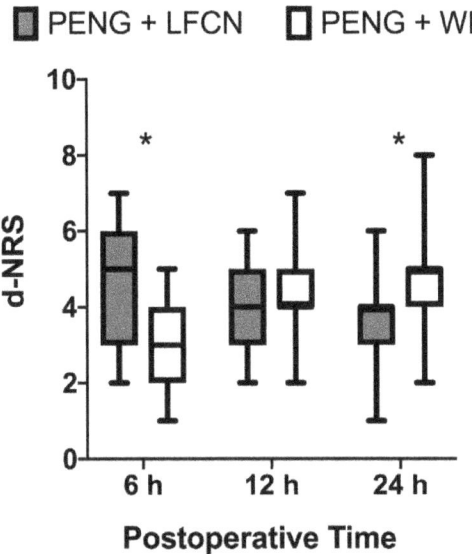

Figure 4. Dynamic postoperative pain. The box plot shows postoperative pain scores in both study groups. Data include dynamic pain reported at three different postoperative time points (6, 12 and 24 h). Pain severity is expressed using a 0–10 numeric rating scale, with 0 equal to no pain and 10 being the worst imaginable pain. Values are expressed as median (horizontal bars) with 25th–75th (box) and range of minimum to maximum value (whiskers); * denotes statistical significance ($p < 0.05$). PENG: pericapsular nerve group block; WI: wound infiltration. LFCN: lateral femoral cutaneous nerve block; d-NRS: numeric rating scale on movement (dynamic).

Secondary outcomes are summarized in Table 2.

Total morphine consumption did not differ among groups, with a mean $\pm$ SD of 6.9 ± 3.6 mg for LCFN vs. 6.5 ± 4.6 for WI ($p = 0.45$). Regarding functional outcomes, the LFCN group showed a worse ROM at 6 h postoperatively ($59.8° \pm 11.2$ vs. $71.4° \pm 15.5$, $p = 0.011$), while a better ROM was noticed at 24 h ($71.4° \pm 15.5$ vs. 60.6 ± 16.5, $p = 0.018$), with no significant differences at 12 h ($69.6° \pm 9.3$ vs. 62.8 ± 12.8, $p = 0.1$).

However, the ability to perform physiotherapy and ambulation during the first POD was comparable between groups, as well as the total length of stay (Table 2).

Moreover, no postoperative quadriceps paralysis was noticed except for one patient in the LFCN group and two patients in the WI group, but in all cases, it occurred only at 6 h postoperatively. Last, the incidence of postoperative complications was comparable and not significant.

Table 2. Secondary outcomes.

	PENG + LFCN (n = 25)	PENG + WI (n = 25)	*p* Value
Morphine Consumption (mg)			
- 24 h	4.3 ± 3.1	3.7 ± 2.9	0.57
- Total	6.9 ± 3.6	6.5 ± 4.6	0.45
Range of Movement (°)			
- 6 h	59.8 ± 11.2	71.4 ± 15.5	0.011
- 12 h	69.6 ± 9.3	62.8 ± 12.8	0.1
- 24 h	71.6 ± 9.9	60.6 ± 16.5	0.018
Quadriceps Paralysis 6/12/24 h, n (%)	1 (4%)/0/0	2 (8%)/0/0	>0.9
Ability to perform physiotherapy at POD1, n (%)	25 (100%)	25 (100%)	>0.9
Ability to ambulation at POD1, n (%)	25 (100%)	24 (96%)	>0.9
Length of stay (days)	2 (2–3)	2 (2–4)	0.96
Nausea/vomiting, n (%)	1 (4%)	2 (8%)	>0.9
Dizziness, n (%)	0	0	-
Vascular Puncture, n (%)	0	0	-

Values are reported as number (percentage) of subjects, mean ± standard deviation (SD) or median and interquartile range (IQR). LFCN: lateral femoral cutaneous nerve block; POD: postoperative day; WI: wound infiltration; PENG: pericapsular nerve group block.

4. Discussion

PENG block, despite being shown to be effective for postoperative analgesia following THA in different randomized clinical trials [14,19–21], is analgesically incomplete, as it does not cover the skin, which has the highest concentration of nociceptors involved in this kind of surgery. For this reason, several trials have investigated combining PENG block with other regional techniques, including periarticular infiltration, intra-articular injection and quadratus lumborum block [22–26].

In our study, both LFCN and WI ensured successful analgesia combined with PENG block, as no severe pain scores were noticed at any time point among the groups, although there were some differences. The WI group showed better analgesia and range of movements at 6 h after surgery compared to the LFCN group, which showed better scores at 24 h postoperatively. However, these differences did not impact opioid consumption or the remaining functional outcomes, including ambulation and physiotherapy. These results lead us to speculate about some clinical considerations, as they may reflect the strength and limitations of both techniques.

LCFN innervates only part of the skin involved in post-surgical pain following THA via the posterior approach, and this could justify the better analgesia in the WI group during the first postoperative hours. In contrast, better pain scores at 24 h postoperatively may be explained by the local anesthetic pharmacokinetics, which are characterized by a slower systemic absorption in the case of perineural rather than subcutaneous administration [27]. Another aspect to discuss is the discrepancy of ROM, which increases over time in the LFCN group, while it decreases in the WI group. As the articular ROM, in the absence of muscular block, may be strictly dependent on analgesia (in an indirectly proportional relationship with pain scores), it is reasonable to think that the inverted trend regarding ROM among the two groups reflects the same tendency of pain scores.

This is the first clinical trial analyzing the effect of PENG block compared to LFCN block or WI for postoperative analgesia after THA.

Gurbuz et al. explored a similar association through a prospective evaluation of 22 patients undergoing total hip replacement. They found a longer time for first analgesic demand in the WI group, although the LFCN group had lower pain scores at 24 h, similar to our study. However this study had important limitations including a lack of randomization, a poor sample size, and the surgical approach was not specified [28]. Dr. Liang and colleagues have recently demonstrated the superiority of PENG block combined with LFCN block vs. supra-inguinal FIB in improving postoperative analgesia after THA [8]. However, the study population was heterogeneous, as both fractured and non-fractured patients were included. Moreover, Dr. Liang compared the association of PENG plus LFCN block vs. SIFI block, which gives an indirect LFCN block itself, and for this reason, it seems unclear if any differences in outcomes can be attributed to the effect of LFCN block rather than PENG block.

Future studies may focus on the combination of PENG block with other techniques to enhance postoperative skin analgesia. In particular, the iliohypogastric nerve and subcostal nerve have been shown to innervate most of the skin involved in surgery, and they could easily be blocked through fascia transversalis or a lateral quadratus lumborum block [5].

At the same time, LFCN block could be added to WI to maximize the analgesic effect of both technique during the first 24 h, as suggested by this study, while being careful about the maximum recommended local anesthetic dosage.

In this study, we used 0.5% ropivacaine in our daily practice. We prefer this concentration to lower ones aiming to enhance block duration, as the rate of LA absorption (which impacts on block's duration) also depends on the administered dosage [27], although no studies have yet analyzed the impact of different ropivacaine dosages on PENG block, LFCN block and WI in hip surgery. Despite a high concentration of ropivacaine, the total dosage administered to every patient (200 mg) was not superior to the maximum dosage recommended for one shot nerve block in adults (250 mg). Moreover, after administration of LA, patients were always monitored to exclude early prodromal symptoms related to Local Anesthetic Systemic Toxicity (LAST), like perioral paresthesia, metallic taste and tinnitus. In addition, clinical and ECG monitoring were maintained until discharge from PACU.

Regarding the duration of the WI analgesic effect, we think it may be prolonged through the use of a continuous technique or liposomal local anesthetics, as already demonstrated in different surgeries [13,29,30].

Last, we would like to discuss three cases (one in the LFCN group and two in the WI group) of postoperative quadriceps paralysis recorded at 6 h.

As described by a recent cadaveric study, this event could be related to the spread of local anesthetic to the femoral nerve during the execution of PENG block, especially when more than 13 mL is injected [31]. However, this has never been demonstrated to cause a significant impact on postoperative functional outcomes, including physiotherapy and ambulation. Not by chance, although Aliste et al. showed a similar incidence of quadriceps paralysis [19], it did not influence functional outcomes, and the same was true for our study. It is worth investigating the use of newer high definition US technology to better identify the optimal injection point and LA spread during the PENG block execution in order to further reduce the risk of femoral nerve involvement.

Limitations

This study has several limitations.

Our actual institutional protocols require the patients to start ambulation after 24 h, and for this reason, it was not possible to investigate the ability of patients to walk before this time point. The same issue regards the ability to start of physiotherapy, which was assessed on POD 1. Future studies assessing these outcomes in earlier time points may overcome these limits.

Secondary outcomes including opioid consumption and length of stay did not show significant differences, although our sample size was powered 90% only for main outcomes: that means higher samples may be required to significantly evaluate the true effect of these outcomes. Moreover, we missed the assessment of other functional outcomes, i.e., the timed up and go (TUG) and walking tests, although its accuracy could be limited by different baseline health statuses and muscular tropisms among patients [32].

Pain scores were recorded only during the first 24 h after surgery, although, based on our clinical experience and our previous study, we consider this time interval to be the most critical for postoperative analgesia following THA via the posterior approach. Furthermore, we did not take the social differences among patients into account, and this could represent a potential bias in pain reporting.

Regarding the assessment of quadriceps strength, we did not use any muscular strength grading to differentiate between paralysis and paresis, as in other studies [19]. However, this method has been shown to have several limitations due to the variability in examiners' subjective perceptions [33].

Our study focused on postoperative acute pain, although it would be interesting for future investigations to analyze the impact of these regional anesthesia techniques on chronic postoperative pain, whose incidence is estimated to be 10% for THA [34]. In this study, we used multimodal analgesia through NSAIDs, which positively impacts postoperative pain and may overestimate the efficacy of a regional anesthesia technique. However, NSAIDs "around the clock" has been applied to both groups at the same dosages, and this is reasonably unlikely to represent a bias.

Lastly, although we monitored clinical and vital signs to exclude LAST, we did not measure systemic absorption rates. Future studies should look at blood levels of ropivacaine after PENG block in order to confirm the safety of this technique and investigate other possible mechanism of actions (systemic?).

5. Conclusions

LFCN block was not inferior to WI for postoperative analgesia and functional recovery in association with PENG block during the first postoperative day, although it had worse short-term pain scores.

However, no significant differences were observed in functional recovery and opioid consumption. Based on these results, it is possible to consider both LFCN block and WI as valuable options to cause skin analgesia after THA. Moreover, we hypothesize that an association of LFCN block and WI combined with PENG block may enhance the analgesic effect of both of the techniques during the first 24 h. However, future studies are expected to confirm this hypothesis and find the best combination between PENG block and other techniques to enhance analgesia and functional outcomes after THA.

Author Contributions: G.P.: conceptualization, methodology, investigation, writing—original draft; F.C.: conceptualization, methodology, investigation; A.S.: data curation, visualization; A.R.: data curation; formal analysis, software; L.M.R.: investigation, data curation; T.L.: investigation, data curation; A.H.: investigation, data curation; F.L.: investigation, data curation; F.G.: investigation, data curation; L.S.: conceptualization, validation, writing—review and editing; A.M.: conceptualization, validation, writing—review and editing; F.E.A.: project administration, supervision; M.C.: conceptualization, resources, supervision; R.C.: writing—review and editing, validation, supervision. All authors have read and agreed to the published version of the manuscript.

Funding: This research received no external funding.

Institutional Review Board Statement: The study protocol has been approved by local institutional ethics committee (protocol number: 34.22, 24 May 2022). The present study has been registered on the public registry clinicaltrials.gov (identifier: NCT05432011). The study was conducted according to the guidelines of the Declaration of Helsinki.

Informed Consent Statement: Informed consent was obtained from all subjects involved in the study.

Data Availability Statement: Data are available upon reasonable request. Please contact the corresponding author (Alessandro Strumia: a.strumia@policlinicocampus.it).

Conflicts of Interest: The authors declare no conflicts of interest.

References

1. Girón-Arango, L.; Peng, P.W.H.; Chin, K.J.; Brull, R.; Perlas, A. Pericapsular Nerve Group (PENG) Block for Hip Fracture. *Reg. Anesth. Pain Med.* **2018**, *43*, 859–863. [CrossRef] [PubMed]
2. Del Buono, R.; Padua, E.; Pascarella, G.; Costa, F.; Tognù, A.; Terranova, G.; Greco, F.; Fajardo Perez, M.; Barbara, E. Pericapsular nerve group block: An overview. *Minerva Anestesiol.* **2021**, *87*, 458–466. [CrossRef] [PubMed]
3. Wang, Y.; Wen, H.; Wang, M.; Lu, M. The Efficiency of Ultrasound-Guided Pericapsular Nerve Group Block for Pain Management after Hip Surgery: A Meta-analysis. *Pain Ther.* **2023**, *12*, 81–92. [CrossRef] [PubMed]
4. Fede, C.; Porzionato, A.; Petrelli, L.; Fan, C.; Pirri, C.; Biz, C.; De Caro, R.; Stecco, C. Fascia and soft tissues innervation in the human hip and their possible role in post-surgical pain. *J. Orthop. Res.* **2020**, *38*, 1646–1654. [CrossRef]
5. Nielsen, T.D.; Moriggl, B.; Barckman, J.; Jensen, J.M.; Kølsen-Petersen, J.A.; Søballe, K.; Børglum, J.; Bendtsen, T.F. Cutaneous anaesthesia of hip surgery incisions with iliohypogastric and subcostal nerve blockade: A randomised trial. *Acta Anaesthesiol. Scand.* **2019**, *63*, 101–110. [CrossRef] [PubMed]
6. Corujo, A.; Franco, C.D.; Williams, J.M. The sensory territory of the lateral cutaneous nerve of the thigh as determined by anatomic dissections and ultrasound-guided blocks. *Reg. Anesth. Pain Med.* **2012**, *37*, 561–564. [CrossRef] [PubMed]
7. Thybo, K.H.; Mathiesen, O.; Dahl, J.B.; Schmidt, H.; Hägi-Pedersen, D. Lateral femoral cutaneous nerve block after total hip arthroplasty: A randomised trial. *Acta Anaesthesiol. Scand.* **2016**, *60*, 1297–1305. [CrossRef] [PubMed]
8. Liang, L.; Zhang, C.; Dai, W.; He, K. Comparison between pericapsular nerve group (PENG) block with lateral femoral cutaneous nerve block and supra-inguinal fascia iliaca compartment block (S-FICB) for total hip arthroplasty: A randomized controlled trial. *J. Anesth.* **2023**, *37*, 503–510. [CrossRef]
9. da Costa, A.O.; Izolani, G.V.; Monteiro de Souza, I.F.; Martins Santiago, B.V. Continuous pericapsular nerve group (PENG) block through an elastomeric infusion system, associated with the lateral cutaneous nerve block of the thigh for total hip arthroplasty. *BMJ Case Rep.* **2022**, *15*, e246833. [CrossRef]
10. Thallaj, A. Combined PENG and LFCN blocks for postoperative analgesia in hip surgery—A case report. *Saudi J. Anaesth.* **2019**, *13*, 381–383. [CrossRef]
11. Marques, E.M.; Blom, A.W.; Lenguerrand, E.; Wylde, V.; Noble, S.M. Local anaesthetic wound infiltration in addition to standard anaesthetic regimen in total hip and knee replacement: Long-term cost-effectiveness analyses alongside the APEX randomised controlled trials. *BMC Med.* **2015**, *13*, 151. [CrossRef] [PubMed]
12. Banerjee, P.; McLean, C. The efficacy of multimodal high-volume wound infiltration in primary total hip replacement. *Orthopedics* **2011**, *34*, e522–e529. [CrossRef] [PubMed]
13. Paladini, G.; Di Carlo, S.; Musella, G.; Petrucci, E.; Scimia, P.; Ambrosoli, A.; Cofini, V.; Fusco, P. Continuous Wound Infiltration of Local Anesthetics in Postoperative Pain Management: Safety, Efficacy and Current Perspectives. *J. Pain Res.* **2020**, *13*, 285–294. [CrossRef] [PubMed]
14. Del Buono, R.; Pascarella, G.; Costa, F.; Terranova, G.; Leoni, M.L.; Barbara, E.; Carassiti, M.; Agrò, F.E. Predicting difficult spinal anesthesia: Development of a neuraxial block assessment score. *Minerva Anestesiol.* **2021**, *87*, 648–654. [CrossRef] [PubMed]
15. Pascarella, G.; Costa, F.; Hazboun, A.; Del Buono, R.; Strumia, A.; Longo, F.; Ruggiero, A.; Schiavoni, L.; Mattei, A.; Cataldo, R.; et al. Ultrasound predictors of difficult spinal anesthesia: A prospective single-blind observational study. *Minerva Anestesiol.* **2023**, *89*, 996–1002. [CrossRef] [PubMed]
16. Pascarella, G.; Costa, F.; Del Buono, R.; Strumia, A.; Cataldo, R.; Agrò, F.E.; Carassiti, M. Defining the optimal spread of local anesthetic during pericapsular nerve group (PENG) block may help to avoid short-term motor block (reply to Aliste et al.). *Reg. Anesth. Pain Med.* **2022**, *47*, 200–201. [CrossRef] [PubMed]
17. Anger, M.; Valovska, T.; Beloeil, H.; Lirk, P.; Joshi, G.P.; Van de Velde, M.; Raeder, J. PROSPECT guideline for total hip arthroplasty: A systematic review and procedure-specific postoperative pain management recommendations. *Anaesthesia* **2021**, *76*, 1082–1097. [CrossRef] [PubMed]
18. Pascarella, G.; Costa, F.; Del Buono, R.; Pulitanò, R.; Strumia, A.; Piliego, C.; De Quattro, E.; Cataldo, R.; Agrò, F.E.; Carassiti, M. Impact of the pericapsular nerve group (PENG) block on postoperative analgesia and functional recovery following total hip arthroplasty: A randomised, observer-masked, controlled trial. *Anaesthesia* **2021**, *76*, 1492–1498. [CrossRef] [PubMed]
19. Aliste, J.; Layera, S.; Bravo, D.; Jara, Á.; Muñoz, G.; Barrientos, C.; Wulf, R.; Brañez, J.; Finlayson, R.J.; Tran, Q. Randomized comparison between pericapsular nerve group (PENG) block and suprainguinal fascia iliaca block for total hip arthroplasty. *Reg. Anesth. Pain Med.* **2021**, *46*, 874–878. [CrossRef]
20. Choi, Y.S.; Park, K.K.; Lee, B.; Nam, W.S.; Kim, D.H. Pericapsular Nerve Group (PENG) Block versus Supra-Inguinal Fascia Iliaca Compartment Block for Total Hip Arthroplasty: A Randomized Clinical Trial. *J. Pers. Med.* **2022**, *12*, 408. [CrossRef]
21. Farag, A.; Hendi, N.I.; Diab, R.A. Does pericapsular nerve group block have limited analgesia at the initial post-operative period? Systematic review and meta-analysis. *J. Anesth.* **2023**, *37*, 138–153. [CrossRef] [PubMed]
22. Lin, D.Y.; Brown, B.; Morrison, C.; Fraser, N.S.; Chooi, C.S.L.; Cehic, M.G.; McLeod, D.H.; Henningsen, M.D.; Sladojevic, N.; Kroon, H.M.; et al. The Pericapsular Nerve Group (PENG) block combined with Local Infiltration Analgesia (LIA) compared to placebo and LIA in hip arthroplasty surgery: A multi-center double-blinded randomized-controlled trial. *BMC Anesthesiol.* **2022**, *22*, 252. [CrossRef]

23. Hu, J.; Wang, Q.; Hu, J.; Kang, P.; Yang, J. Efficacy of Ultrasound-Guided Pericapsular Nerve Group (PENG) Block Combined With Local Infiltration Analgesia on Postoperative Pain after Total Hip Arthroplasty: A Prospective, Double-Blind, Randomized Controlled Trial. *J. Arthroplast.* **2023**, *38*, 1096–1103. [CrossRef]
24. Et, T.; Korkusuz, M. Comparison of pericapsular nerve group (peng) block with intra-articular and quadratus lumborum block in primary total hip arthroplasty: A randomized controlled trial. *Korean J. Anesthesiol.* **2023**, *76*, 575–585. [CrossRef]
25. Zheng, J.; Pan, D.; Zheng, B.; Ruan, X. Preoperative pericapsular nerve group (PENG) block for total hip arthroplasty: A randomized, placebo-controlled trial. *Reg. Anesth. Pain Med.* **2022**, *47*, 155–160. [CrossRef]
26. Bravo, D.; Aliste, J.; Layera, S.; Fernández, D.; Erpel, H.; Aguilera, G.; Arancibia, H.; Barrientos, C.; Wulf, R.; León, S.; et al. Randomized clinical trial comparing pericapsular nerve group (PENG) block and periarticular local anesthetic infiltration for total hip arthroplasty. *Reg. Anesth. Pain Med.* **2023**, *48*, 489–494. [CrossRef] [PubMed]
27. Taylor, A.; McLeod, G. Basic pharmacology of local anaesthetics. *BJA Educ.* **2020**, *20*, 34–41. [CrossRef]
28. Gurbuz, H.; Okmen, K.; Gultekin, A. Postoperative pain management in patients with coxarthrosis undergoing total hip arthroplasty: PENG block combined with LFCN block or wound infiltration? *Minerva Anestesiol.* **2021**, *87*, 1154–1155. [CrossRef] [PubMed]
29. Fusco, P.; Cofini, V.; Petrucci, E.; Scimia, P.; Fiorenzi, M.; Paladini, G.; Behr, A.U.; Borghi, B.; Flamini, S.; Pizzoferrato, R.; et al. Continuous wound infusion and local infiltration analgesia for postoperative pain and rehabilitation after total hip arthroplasty. *Minerva Anestesiol.* **2018**, *84*, 556–564. [CrossRef]
30. Ma, T.T.; Wang, Y.H.; Jiang, Y.F.; Peng, C.B.; Yan, C.; Liu, Z.G.; Xu, W.X. Liposomal bupivacaine versus traditional bupivacaine for pain control after total hip arthroplasty: A meta-analysis. *Medicine* **2017**, *96*, e7190. [CrossRef]
31. Leurcharusmee, P.; Kantakam, P.; Intasuwan, P.; Malatong, Y.; Maikong, N.; Navic, P.; Kitcharanant, N.; Mahakkanukrauh, P.; Tran, Q. Cadaveric study investigating the femoral nerve-sparing volume for pericapsular nerve group (PENG) block. *Reg. Anesth. Pain Med.* **2023**, *48*, 549–552. [CrossRef] [PubMed]
32. Kear, B.M.; Guck, T.P.; McGaha, A.L. Timed Up and Go (TUG) Test: Normative Reference Values for Ages 20 to 59 Years and Relationships With Physical and Mental Health Risk Factors. *J. Prim. Care Community Health* **2017**, *8*, 9–13. [CrossRef] [PubMed]
33. Naqvi, U.; Sherman, A.L. Muscle Strength Grading. In *StatPearls*; StatPearls Publishing LLC.: Treasure Island, FL, USA, 2023.
34. Wylde, V.; Sayers, A.; Lenguerrand, E.; Gooberman-Hill, R.; Pyke, M.; Beswick, A.D.; Dieppe, P.; Blom, A.W. Preoperative widespread pain sensitization and chronic pain after hip and knee replacement: A cohort analysis. *Pain* **2015**, *156*, 47–54. [CrossRef] [PubMed]

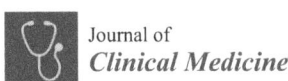

Article

Efficacy and Safety of Magnesium Sulfate as an Adjunct to Ropivacaine Wound Infiltration in Thyroid Surgery: A Prospective, Double-Blind, Randomized Controlled Trial

Stiliani Laskou [1,*], Georgia Tsaousi [2], Chryssa Pourzitaki [3], Georgios Papazisis [3], Isaak Kesisoglou [1] and Konstantinos Sapalidis [1]

1   3rd Surgical Department, School of Medicine, Aristotle University of Thessaloniki, 1st St. Kiriakidi Str, 54636 Thessaloniki, Greece; ikesis@hotmail.com (I.K.); sapalidiskonstantinos@gmail.com (K.S.)
2   Clinic of Anesthesiology and Intensive Care, School of Medicine, Aristotle University of Thessaloniki, 54124 Thessaloniki, Greece; tsaousig@otenet.gr
3   Department of Clinical Pharmacology, Faculty of Medicine, School of Health Sciences, Aristotle University of Thessaloniki, 54006 Thessaloniki, Greece; chpour@gmail.com (C.P.); papazisg@auth.gr (G.P.)
*   Correspondence: stelaskou@gmail.com

Citation: Laskou, S.; Tsaousi, G.; Pourzitaki, C.; Papazisis, G.; Kesisoglou, I.; Sapalidis, K. Efficacy and Safety of Magnesium Sulfate as an Adjunct to Ropivacaine Wound Infiltration in Thyroid Surgery: A Prospective, Double-Blind, Randomized Controlled Trial. *J. Clin. Med.* 2024, 13, 4499. https://doi.org/10.3390/jcm13154499

Academic Editors: Giustino Varrassi, Felice Eugenio Agro, Giuseppe Pascarella and Fabio Costa

Received: 10 June 2024
Revised: 18 July 2024
Accepted: 27 July 2024
Published: 1 August 2024

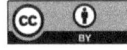
Abstract: Background/Objective: Wound infiltration with local anesthetics emerges as a promising modality for postoperative pain alleviation. However, such strategies in neck surgery have not been a well-established practice. To assess wound infiltration with ropivacaine plus magnesium sulfate for pain relief following thyroid surgery. **Methods**: This prospective, double-blind, randomized study enrolled 68 patients who underwent thyroid surgery. Concerning the solution used for surgical wound infiltration, the study participants were randomly allocated into three groups: (1) 100 mg of ropivacaine (Group R); (2) 100 mg of ropivacaine plus magnesium sulfate 10 mg/kg (Group RMg); and (3) normal saline which served as a placebo (Group P). Pain perception both at rest and at movement, was measured using the Visual Analogue Scale (VAS) at 30 min, as well as at 1, 2, 4, 6, 12, and 24 h postoperatively. The total consumption of analgesics in morphine equivalents was also recorded. Moreover, adverse effects and patient satisfaction were recorded. Cortisol, TNF-α, and IL-6 levels were measured 30 min before infiltration and 6 h and 24 h postoperatively. **Results**: Demographics and clinical characteristics were similar between the groups. The VAS scores at rest and during movement were significantly lower in the RMg group compared to the saline or ropivacaine groups. Total analgesic consumption was also significantly lower in the RMg group. No operation-, wound-, or infiltration-related adverse effects were recorded in the study groups. Better overall satisfaction was obtained for the RMg group. **Conclusions**: Ropivacaine plus magnesium sulfate wound infiltration provided better pain control and the analgesic effect was more significant, contributing to effective postoperative analgesia in patients undergoing thyroid surgery.

Keywords: ropivacaine; magnesium sulfate; postoperative pain; analgesia; thyroidectomy

1. Introduction

Thyroid surgery represents a common operation with approximately 93,000 thyroidectomies being performed in the United States each year, while parathyroidectomy is comparatively rare, as the incidence of primary hyperparathyroidism is approximately 25 cases per 100,000 [1].

Postoperative pain related to thyroid or parathyroid surgery can be a major challenge for patient care. Pain control after thyroid surgery improves patients' quality of life and allows a quick return to normal daily activities. Adequate postoperative pain control is customarily managed by a broad spectrum of analgesics, including nonsteroidal anti-inflammatory drugs (NSAIDs) or opioid analgesics, which constitute the top analgesic choices [2,3]. Yet, both regimens are frequently linked to adverse effects.

Local wound infiltration has long been used in general surgery to reduce postoperative pain intensity and minimize the need for analgesics. Evidence indicates that thyroidectomy wound infiltration constitutes an easy-to-implement technique performed by the surgeon himself, while it elongates the time frame until rescue analgesia [4]. In the current clinical practice, magnesium sulfate is widely applied in the perioperative setting for its multifactorial properties, among which it has been shown to mitigate analgesic requirements [5–8]. Relevant reports indicate that the implementation of wound infiltration with magnesium sulfate and ropivacaine mixture seems to reduce postoperative tramadol requirements after radical prostatectomy [5–8].

To the authors' knowledge, no studies exist in the current literature investigating the use of magnesium sulfate as an adjunct to local anesthetics for wound infiltration thyroidectomy/parathyroidectomy. Thus, the present study aims to evaluate the effectiveness of wound infiltration with ropivacaine plus magnesium sulfate mixture for postoperative pain control in patients undergoing thyroid or parathyroid surgery, with the safety of this practice constituting the secondary study endpoint.

2. Materials and Methods

2.1. General Information

After institutional approval was obtained from the Ethics Committee of the School of Medicine of Aristotle University of Thessaloniki (No. 3.468/18-1-2022), all consecutive adult patients of both sexes and the American Society of Anesthesiologists (ASA) classification I–II, scheduled for thyroidectomy/parathyroidectomy from January 2022 to January 2024, were eligible for enrolment in this study. This study was conducted following the Declaration of Helsinki guidelines, while written informed consent was obtained from all patients before study enrollment. The trial was registered in the ClinicalTrials.gov database with the unique reference ID NCT05294393.

The exclusion criteria included the indication for selective lateral neck dissection, previous cervical operation, long-term analgesic drug use, known or suspected allergy to local anesthetics, and a major complication of surgery or anesthesia (major bleeding, allergy to anesthetic products).

2.2. Randomization and Masking

Patients were allocated to three groups using a computer randomization list (www.sealedenvelope.com, assessed on 19 January 2022) developed by a person irrelevant to the study protocol. Permuted block randomization was performed using a random number table with equal allocation and a block size of 6. An anesthesia nurse, being unaware of the study protocol, prepared an unlabeled syringe of 15 mL solution, including normal saline which served as a placebo (Group P), ropivacaine 100 mg (Group R), or a mixture of 100 mg ropivacaine plus 10 mg/kg magnesium sulfate (Group RMg). The patients, operating team, and investigator who served as the outcome assessor were blinded to the infiltrated solution.

2.3. Anesthesia and Surgical Procedure

A standardized protocol was applied to all patients. The same anesthesia and surgical team were involved in all procedures. Preoperatively, all patients were premedicated with 0.5 mg alprazolam. In the operating room, venous access with an 18–20 G IV cannula and standard hemodynamic monitoring were applied to all patients. After preoxygenation with 100% oxygen for 3 min, anesthesia induction was established by intravenous 2–2.5 mg·kg^{-1} propofol, 0.2 mg·kg^{-1} cis-atracurium, and target-controlled infusion (TCI) of remifentanil (3 mcg·mL^{-1}). Endotracheal intubation was facilitated by spiral endotracheal tubes with inner diameters of 7.5 and 8 mm for females and males, respectively. After anesthesia induction, 8 mg dexamethasone and 40 mg omeprazole were also administered. Maintenance of anesthesia was ensured with desflurane, while remifentanil in TCI mode was applied for intraoperative analgesia. Desflurane was used for its rapid onset and offset, enabling the swift and smooth awakening of the involved patients. A change of 20% in heart rate or mean blood pressure guided TCI rate alterations.

Patients were placed in the supine position on the operating table, with the neck hyperextended. Through a 4–7 cm skin incision (depending on the size of the thyroid), subplatysmal flaps were created, and strap muscles were separated in the midline and reflected laterally. The middle, superior, and inferior thyroid vessels were then divided. The same steps were repeated for the removal of the contralateral lobe. After complete hemostasis and before wound closure, the surgeon, blinded to the applied medications, soaked a pad with the solution over the anterior face of the trachea, then infiltrated, using a 21-gauge needle, the strap muscles and subcutaneous tissues in both flaps as well as the surgical edges. Extra attention was paid to avoid laryngeal nerve infiltration and thus preserve laryngeal function after surgery. Before surgical wound closure, all patients received 1 g of paracetamol and 4 mg of ondansetron.

Finally, the wound was closed using interrupted 3-0 and 4-0 polyglactin sutures to approximate the strap muscles and the platysma layer, respectively. The skin was closed with 4-0 interrupted polypropylene sutured. Suction drains were not used. All patients were extubated after ensuring enough muscle strength and the ability to follow all commands. Surgical time (incision to wound closure) and awakening time (anesthesia discontinuation to tracheal extubation) were also registered for each participant.

2.4. Assessment of Postoperative Pain

All patients were familiarized with a 10 cm Visual Analogue Scale (VAS) preoperatively for pain intensity evaluation. All study participants were followed for 24 h for pain evaluation and adverse effect occurrence. The VAS score at rest and during movement was recorded at 30 min and at 1, 2, 4, 6, 12, and 24 h after surgery completion. In cases of moderate pain at rest (VAS score > 4), 1 gr paracetamol was administered as a rescue analgesic drug, while in cases of severe pain (VAS score > 6), 40 mg parecoxib or 50–100 mg tramadol was administered targeting a VAS < 4. Total analgesic requirements up to 24 h postoperatively were calculated in oral morphine equivalents. Blood samples for the determination of cortisol, TNF-α, and IL-6 levels were collected 30 min before surgical wound infiltration and at 6 and 24 h after surgery completion. Blood samples were placed in dry tubes and centrifuged within 5 min of collection. Thereafter, plasma serum was separated and stored at $-70\,^\circ$C until analyzed. Patient satisfaction was also evaluated with a 5-point scale upon hospital discharge.

2.5. Outcomes

The primary study outcome was total analgesic consumption up to 24 h after the study completion. The time to the first analgesic request, pain intensity assessed by the VAS at the predefined time points, magnitude of the inflammatory response, occurrence of adverse effects, and patient satisfaction constituted secondary study endpoints.

2.6. Statistical Analysis

Based on the findings of previous relevant clinical studies in patients undergoing lumbar laminectomy, a sample size of 19 patients was used for each group, with a two-sided alpha of 0.05 and a power of 80% to detect a 24 h reduction in the consumption of rescue analgesics (in oral morphine equivalents) by 30% (standard deviation of 15) between tested groups. Allowing for a 20% drop-out rate, the final study population was set at 68 patients. The sample size analysis was conducted using MedCalc version 16.1.

Data normality was assessed by the Kolmogorov–Smirnoff test. Friedman's non-parametric test was applied for continuous variable comparisons over different time points (VAS scores at rest and movement), while pairwise comparisons were achieved by the Durbin–Conover test (24 h analgesic consumption). Comparisons by group for each time point were performed by the Kruskal–Wallis test, while the Dwass–Steel–Critchlow–Fligner test was used for pair comparison. Cross-tabulations were applied for qualitative variable comparisons. Data of inflammatory markers were normalized by inverse normal transformation through their fractional rank to facilitate the use of a parametric test. A mixed ANOVA analysis was performed. The sphericity testing criterion with the Mauchly test was not met ($p < 0.05$) and a Greenhouse–Geisser correction was applied. The equality of variances test for equality of covariance in the three patient groups indicated equality of variances at all time points.

The SPSS package (version 29.0) was used for statistical analysis, while a p-value < 0.05 was considered statistically significant.

3. Results

3.1. Clinical and Demographic Characteristics of Study Patients

From the total of 68 patients initially stratified in this study, two were excluded due to reoperation for severe bleeding control, leaving 66 patients for the final analysis (Figure 1). Demographics and intraoperative data were comparable between study groups (Table 1). There was no statistically significant difference between the groups. As far as the type of surgery was concerned, 41 thyroidectomies were performed for multinodular disease, seven for toxic goiter, six for carcinoma, five for concurrent hyperparathyroidism and goiter, and seven for hyperparathyroidism.

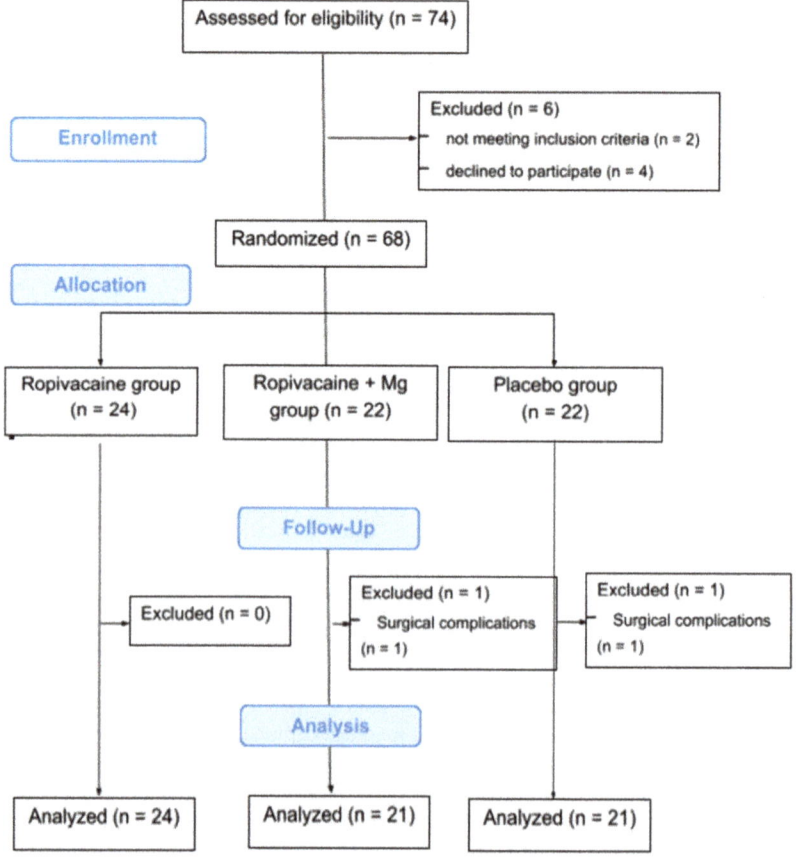

Figure 1. CONSORT diagram. Notes: R, ropivacaine; RMg, ropivacaine plus magnesium sulfate; P, placebo.

Table 1. Demographic and intraoperative characteristics of the patients in the ropivacaine (R), ropivacaine plus magnesium sulfate (RMg), and placebo (P) groups. NOTES: R, ropivacaine; RMg, ropivacaine plus magnesium sulphate; P, placebo; M, male; F, female; kg/m^2, kilogram per square meter; cm, centimeter; µg, microgram; min, minute.

	Group R	Group RMg	Group P
Sex (M:F)	4:20	5:16	5:16
Age (years) BMI (kg/m^2)	54.78 ± 15.08	51.48 ± 15.56	62.14 ± 10.29
BMI (kg/m^2)	27.49 ± 4.44	28.06 ± 6.25	27.52 ± 5.70
Hamilton Anxiety Scale	13.17 ± 5.44	14.05 ± 4.19	12.86 ± 3.55
Duration of Surgery (min)	108.54 ± 38.16	123.52 ± 27.11	125.05 ± 32.23
Anesthesia Interruption to Extubation Time (min)	5.75 ± 1.87	6.19 ± 3.37	6.43 ± 2.40
Incision Length (cm)	4.39 ± 1.05	4.50 ± 0.62	4.54 ± 0.72
Remifentanil TCI (µg)	795.96 ± 287.16	729.96 ± 389.40	1064.36 ± 457.94

3.2. Total Analgesic Requirements

The total dose of analgesics administered over the 24 h postoperative period varied significantly between the three groups. Patients in Group RMg received less total analgesic requirements than in Group R (7.53 ± 14.55 mg vs. 18.30 ± 13.16 mg, $p < 0.01$, respectively). Patients in the placebo group showed higher analgesic demand than in the RMg and R groups (39.35 ± 19.93 mg vs. 7.53 ± 14.55 mg vs. 18.30 ± 13.16 mg, $p < 0.001$).

Patients in Group P received their first analgesic drug within the first postoperative hour, while the time to first analgesic request was significantly elongated in the R and RMg groups (Table 2). The time for analgesic demand was significantly lower in the RMg group compared to other groups and in Group R compared to the placebo (χ^2 (2,66) = 29.42, $p < 0.001$).

Table 2. Time to first analgesic request and analgesic consumption expressed in morphine equivalents.

	Group R	Group RMg	Group P
1st analgesic requirement (min)	140.60 ± 127.56 *	184.13 ± 131.58 *^	53.75 ± 60.62
Total analgesic requirements in morphine equivalents (mg)	18.30 ± 13.16 *	7.53 ± 14.55 *^	39.35 ± 19.93

Notes: * $p < 0.001$ between treatment groups vs. control. ^ $p < 0.01$ between Mg and RMg groups.

3.3. Pain Evaluation

The VAS score at rest of all study patients decreased after thyroidectomy at all time points. Higher pain intensity was observed during the first two postoperative hours. Statistical significance was noted when comparing the 1st to 2nd, 4th to 6th, and 6th to 8th postoperative hours.

Comparison between groups revealed significant differences at all timeframes (χ^2 (6) = 126.34, $p < 0.001$). Analysis showed that the R group obtained lower VAS scores than the placebo at all time intervals. It was also revealed that when magnesium was added to the mixture, the analgesic effect was notably improved compared to ropivacaine alone or the placebo at all time points (Figure 2).

Comparison between groups revealed significant differences at all timeframes (χ^2 (6) = 133.10, $p < 0.001$); ropivacaine showed lower VAS scores compared with the placebo). However, when magnesium was added in the mixture, the analgesic effect was significantly improved. Group RMg showed the lowest VAS scores at all timeframes followed by Group R (Figure 3).

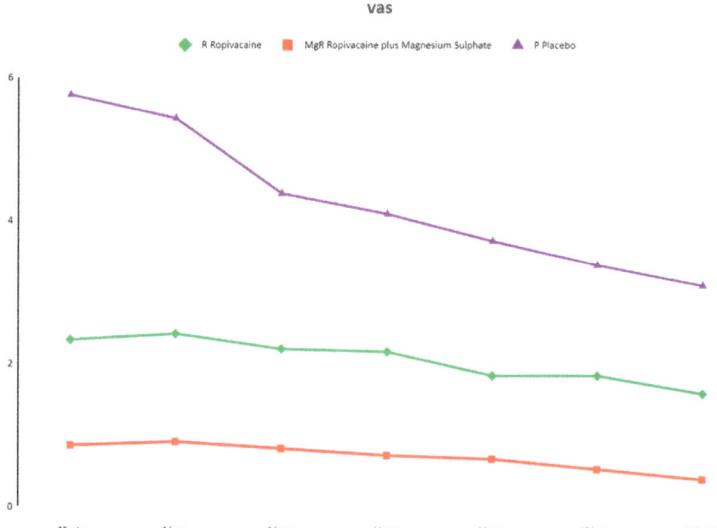

Figure 2. Postoperative Visual Analog Score (VAS) at rest of the three groups presented as the mean and standard deviation. NOTES: All non-parametric Dwass–Steel–Critchlow–Fligner pairwise comparisons were statistically significant at a $p < 0.001$ level. The VAS score at movement of all study patients was increased during the first postoperative hour and decreased afterwards. Statistical significance was noted except for when comparing the 30 min results to the 1st and 2nd h, 2nd to 4th h, and 12th to 24th h.

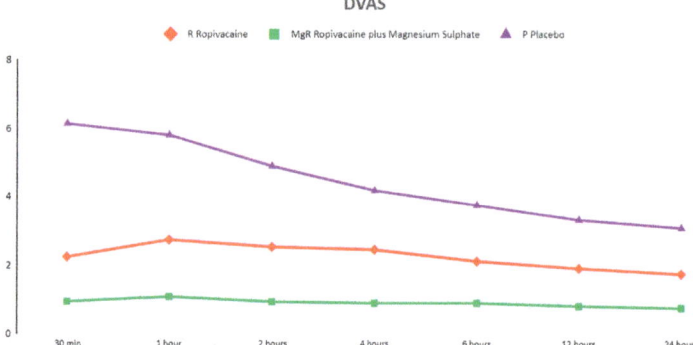

Figure 3. Postoperative Visual Analog Score during movement (DVAS) of the three groups presented as the mean and standard deviation. NOTES: All non-parametric Dwass–Steel–Critchlow–Fligner pairwise comparisons were statistically significant at a $p < 0.001$ level.

3.4. Inflammatory Marker Release

No statistically significant difference between groups was detected for cortisol, IL-6, and TNF-a levels (Figure 4a–c).

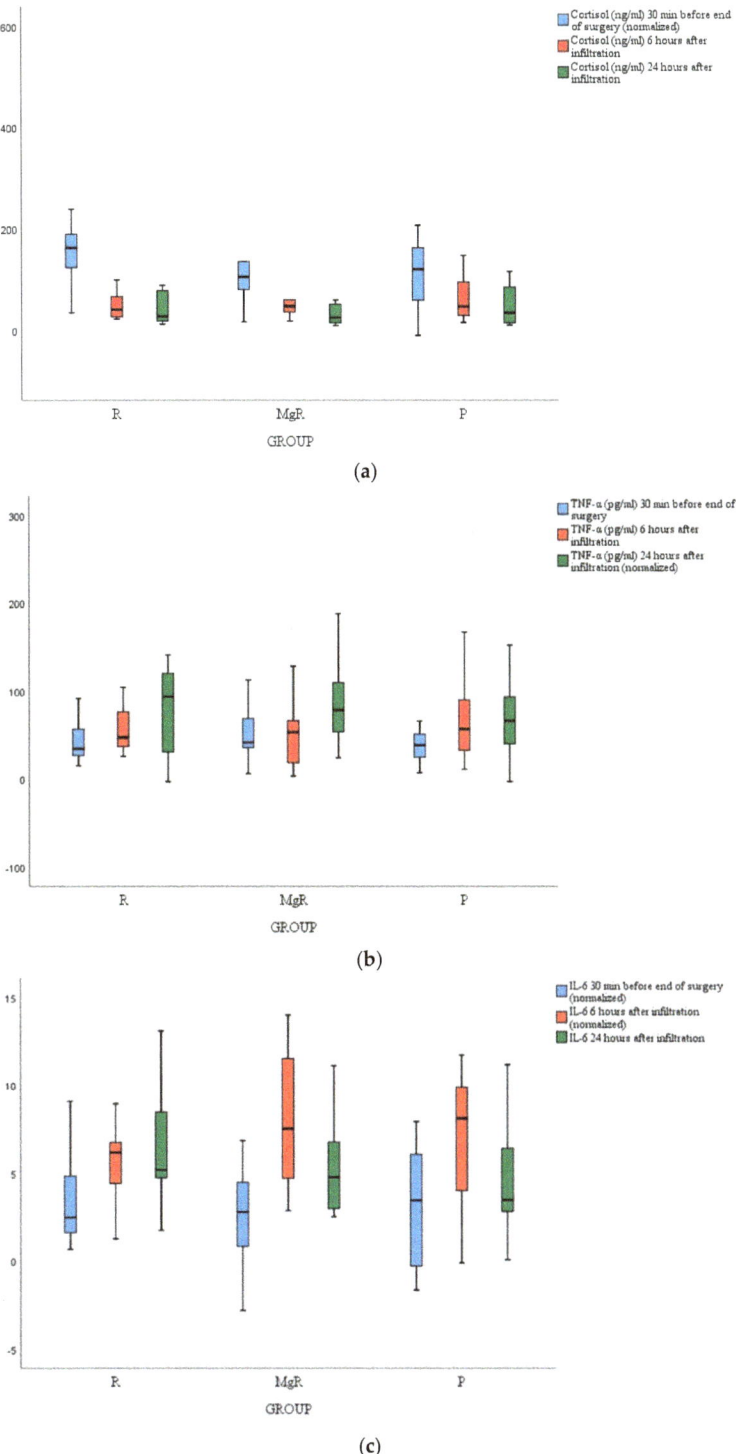

Figure 4. (**a**) Cortisol serum concentration at each time point of assessment; (**b**) TNF-α serum concentration at each time point of assessment; (**c**) IL-6 serum concentration at each time point of assessment.

3.5. Postoperative Complications

A sore throat was the most commonly reported adverse effect, yet no between-group difference was detected. However, the incidences of nausea and vomiting were similar between the treatment groups (Table 3).

Table 3. Postoperative complications. NOTES: PONV, postoperative nausea and vomiting.

	Group R	Group RMg	Group P
PONV	2 (3.3%)	2 (3.3%)	3 (4.9%)
Shiver	1 (6.1%)	1 (1.5%)	0 (0%)
Cough	4 (6.1%)	2 (3%)	2 (3%)
Sore Throat	9 (13.6%)	6 (9.1%)	9 (13.6%)

No immediate or short-term cases of mortality were encountered, while wound complications at the injection sites were absent in the study group. Regarding local infiltration agents, no patient developed complications after infiltration.

3.6. Patients' Satisfaction

Based on the median overall satisfaction score based on a 5-point scale, pairwise comparisons revealed a statistically significant difference (chi-square $(2,66) = 16.00$, $p < 0.001$). Patients in Group RMg (5(1)) reported better overall satisfaction than patients in the placebo group (3 (1.5)), while a marginal statistical difference was found between patients in the R group (4, (1.75)) and patients in the RMg group.

4. Discussion

Postoperative discomfort following thyroid surgery is elicited by multiple causes. Incisional pain especially in the first postoperative day is the major component of this discomfort [9]. The complexity of surgical maneuvers, odynophagia due to endotracheal intubation, and neck soreness caused by the hyperextension position are also incriminated [10]. In the context of Enhanced Recovery After Surgery (ERAS) protocols, which aim to reduce the hospital length of stay while providing faster recovery and functional restoration of the patient, the implementation of a structured analgesic protocol is of paramount importance [11,12].

Pain after thyroid surgery is poorly assessed by many physicians, misjudging the small incision. Although these procedures are characterized by a short duration, surgery-related pain is maximized one hour postoperatively and starts to decline 3 h later [11]. Postoperative pain may delay the patient's discharge as well as return to everyday life.

Pain relief is most commonly achieved by administering NSAIDs and/or opioid analgesics. However, NSAIDs have been associated with potential cardiovascular events, postoperative bleeding, and renal impairment [13]. Meanwhile, opioids are linked to side effects such as sedation, dizziness, nausea, vomiting, constipation, physical dependence, tolerance, and respiratory depression [14].

Based on the fact that the main innervation of the thyroidectomy field originates from the superficial branches of the cervical plexus, regional techniques such as local anesthesia and bilateral superficial and/or deep cervical plexus block could represent a promising method. Local wound infiltration bears the advantage of being a safe and easy-to-implement procedure. It seems that thyroidectomy wound infiltration elongates the timeframe until rescue analgesia. Local anesthetics used for thyroidectomy wound infiltration include the amides bupivacaine, lidocaine, and ropivacaine [9].

In our trial, we tried to achieve a long-lasting infiltrative technique by supplementing ropivacaine with magnesium sulfate. Magnesium sulfate reduces NMDA's receptor binding capacity, preventing central sensitization to a peripheral pain stimulus while preventing the established hyperalgesia [14]. It is even hypothesized to antagonize opioid-induced hyperalgesia as the analgesic effect appears to be better when remifentanil is administered in the anesthetic protocol rather than desflurane [15]. The effects of magnesium sulfate on postoperative pain and opioid consumption have been studied in recent years in a variety of surgical procedures. It has been administered by various routes, including oral, intravenous, intrathecal, and epidural.

Regarding wound infiltration, magnesium sulfate has been applied, alone or as an adjunct, to prostatectomy, caesarian section, lumbar discectomy, and inguinal hernia repair procedures. In laparoscopic prostatectomy cases, wound infiltration with magnesium achieved a superior analgesic effect compared to the placebo, while in inguinal hernia repair, magnesium was less effective compared to local anesthetic infiltration at reducing opioid requirements [15,16]. Similarly, in pediatric adenectomy, the combination of magnesium with levobupivacaine or ropivacaine reduced postoperative pain and the incidence of laryngospasm compared to the administration of levobupivacaine or ropivacaine alone [17,18]. However, different results were obtained by Sun et al. They assumed that the addition of epinephrine to their solution masked the analgesic effect of magnesium [19].

Notably, in lumbar discectomy procedures, a superior nociceptive effect was attributed to the combined administration of ropivacaine or bupivacaine plus magnesium sulfate [20,21]. More recently, Dave et al. applied the combination of bupivacaine and magnesium sulfate in rectal procedures [22]. Such operations require a deep level of anesthesia since the anorectal region is innervated from both the autonomic nervous system and the animal nervous system, while postoperatively, patients experience severe pain and discomfort. It was found that during the first 24 h, combined administration led to superior results in terms of pain management, less opioid consumption, and pain during defecation.

The supplementary use of magnesium sulfate in periarticular injection drug mixtures after total arthroplasty procedures has also provided promising findings in terms of early postoperative pain control [23,24]. Noteworthy enough is that no adverse effect was observed in any of the local infiltration studies with magnesium sulfate.

Ropivacaine is a long-acting amide local anesthetic, which reversibly binds and inactivates sodium channels in the open state, inhibiting sodium ion influx in nerve fibers and blocking the propagation of action potentials. Compared to other local anesthetics, it is less likely to penetrate large myelinated motor fibers, acting selectively on the nociceptive A, B, and C fibers. Manufactured as a pure $S(-)$ enantiomer, it is characterized by significantly less cardiotoxicity and neurotoxicity [25,26].

Thyroidectomy wound infiltration with ropivacaine has been studied in a few randomized clinical trials. Motamed et al. [27] compared thyroidectomy wound infiltration at the end of surgery with ropivacaine vs. placebo and they observed a significant reduction in pain scales as well as opioid consumption during the patient's stay in the recovery room but not in the ward. Their observation was attributed to the low ropivacaine dose (20 mg) used for wound infiltration. Comparing local infiltration with ropivacaine (75 mg), bupivacaine (50 mg), and a placebo, Ayman et al. [11] observed a reduction in postoperative pain with ropivacaine but not with bupivacaine. This effect, however, was significant only during the first postoperative hour [11]. Contrary to previous findings, Miu et al. [9] could not prove any significant analgesic benefit with ropivacaine infiltration (75 mg) or a placebo at the end of thyroid surgery.

It appears that the efficacy of ropivacaine is present but limited when given alone. Both the efficacy and the duration of the method depend on the surgical incision length, as well as the topical agent used [4]. In the same clinical setting, the use of NSAIDs as adjuncts to ropivacaine infiltration promoted an enhanced analgesic effect [12,25,28].

In the present study, we attempted to evaluate the analgesic efficacy of the tested infiltrative agents by assessing the magnitude of the inflammatory markers' release, namely cortisol, TNF-α, and IL-6, but we failed to detect any notable difference between study groups. A plausible explanation for this finding could be the fact that inflammatory response modulation was a secondary study endpoint, and presumably, our study was underpowered for this effect. Over and above, it appears that thyroidectomy-induced stress response is trivial considering that the average VAS score at rest and movement was maintained at clinically acceptable levels throughout the study course [9,29,30].

Several limitations could be acknowledged in the present study. First, a possible drawback could be the absence of serum magnesium level determination, as well as the recording of subsequent magnesium-related adverse effects. Second, intraoperative opioid titration was guided by hemodynamic alterations. Although the implementation of nociception monitoring seems to reflect intraoperative stimuli slightly better than traditionally used parameters and contribute to the quantification of the patient's physiological pain response, to date, none among the commercially available devices has shown a convincing and clinically relevant benefit for its routine use [31–35].

Third, although we applied a randomization process in our study methodology, a higher intraoperative remifentanil consumption was recorded in the placebo group, yet the difference was not statistically significant. This finding could imply the development of a hyperalgesic effect in this group of patients. Fourth, pain assessment was achieved by a subjective scale which could be associated with bias since patients may have interpreted a sore throat or neck pain as incisional pain. Lastly, by conducting a single-center study, our findings reflect the effect of this practice in a defined population subjected to a standardized surgical practice.

5. Conclusions

In conclusion, local wound infiltration with magnesium sulfate as an adjunct to ropivacaine can enhance the postoperative analgesic effect in comparison to either ropivacaine or a placebo following total thyroidectomy, further demonstrating an advanced safety profile. Future large-scale studies are mandatory to enlighten the role of magnesium sulfate as an adjunct analgesic regimen for wound infiltration in this clinical setting.

Author Contributions: S.L., data curation and writing—original draft; G.T., writing—review and editing and formal analysis; C.P., formal analysis; G.P., validation; I.K., resources; K.S., supervision and project administration. All authors have read and agreed to the published version of the manuscript.

Funding: This research received no external funding.

Institutional Review Board Statement: This study was conducted in accordance with the Declaration of Helsinki and approved by the Institutional Review Board (or Ethics Committee) of Aristotle University of Thessaloniki (18.01.2022/3.468).

Informed Consent Statement: Written informed consent was obtained from the patients to publish this paper.

Data Availability Statement: The original contributions presented in the study are included in the article, further inquiries can be directed to the corresponding author.

Conflicts of Interest: The authors declare no conflicts of interest.

References

1. Terris, D.J.; Snyder, S.; Carneiro-Pla, D.; Iii, W.B.I.; Kandil, E.; Orloff, L.; Shindo, M.; Tufano, R.P.; Tuttle, R.M.; Urken, M.; et al. American Thyroid Association statement on outpatient thyroidectomy. *Thyroid* **2013**, *23*, 1193–1202. [CrossRef]
2. Bianchini, C.; Malago, M.; Crema, L.; Aimoni, C.; Matarazzo, T.; Bortolazzi, S.; Ciorba, A.; Pelucchi, S.; Pastore, A. Post-operative pain management in head and neck cancer patients: Predictive factors and efficacy of therapy. *Acta Otorhinolaryngol. Ital.* **2016**, *36*, 91. [CrossRef]
3. Nabata, K.J.; Guo, R.; Nguyen, A.; Osborn, J.A.; Wiseman, S.M. Superiority of non-opioid postoperative pain management after thyroid and parathyroid operations: A systematic review and meta-analysis. *Surg. Oncol.* **2022**, *41*, 101731. [CrossRef]
4. Laskou, S.; Tsaousi, G.; Pourzitaki, C.; Loukipoudi, L.; Papazisis, G.; Kesisoglou, I.; Sapalidis, K. Local Wound Infiltration for Thyroidectomized Patients in the Era of Multimodal Analgesia. *Medicina (Kaunas)* **2023**, *59*, 1662. [CrossRef] [PubMed] [PubMed Central]
5. Tauzin-Fin, P.; Sesay, M.; Svartz, L.; Krol-Houdek, M.C.; Maurette, P. Wound infiltration with magnesium sulphate and ropivacaine mixture reduces postoperative tramadol requirements after radical prostatectomy. *Acta Anaesthesiol. Scand.* **2009**, *53*, 464–469. [CrossRef] [PubMed]

6. Eldaba, A.A.; Amr, Y.M.; Sobhy, R.A. Effect of wound infiltration with bupivacaine or lower dose bupivacaine/magnesium versus placebo for postoperative analgesia after cesarean section. *Anesth. Essays Res.* **2013**, *7*, 336–340.
7. Kundra, S.; Singh, R.M.; Singh, G.; Singh, T.; Jarewal, V.; Katyal, S. Efficacy of Magnesium Sulphate as an Adjunct to Ropivacaine in Local Infiltration for Postoperative Pain Following Lower Segment Caesarean Section. *J. Clin. Diagn. Res.* **2016**, *10*, 18–22. [CrossRef]
8. Donadi, P.; Moningi, S.; Gopinath, R. Comparison of bupivacaine anδ bupivacaine plus magnesium sulphate infiltration for postoperative analgesia in patients undergoing lumbar laminectomy: A prospective randomised double-blinded controlled study. *J. Neuroanaesth. Crit. Care* **2014**, *1*, 183–187.
9. Miu, M.; Royer, C.; Gaillat, C.; Schaup, B.; Menegaux, F.; Langeron, O.; Riou, B.; Aubrun, F. Lack of Analgesic Effect Induced by Ropivacaine Wound Infiltration in Thyroid Surgery: A Randomized, Double-Blind, Placebo-Controlled Trial. *Anesth. Analg.* **2016**, *122*, 559–564. [CrossRef]
10. Lacoste, L.; Thomas, D.; Kraimps, J.L.; Chabin, M.; Ingrand, P.; Barbier, J.; Fusciardi, J. Postthyroidectomy analgesia: Morphine, buprenorphine, or bupivacaine? *J. Clin. Anesth.* **1997**, *9*, 189–193. [CrossRef]
11. Ayman, M.; Materazzi, G.; Bericotti, M.; Rago, R.; Nidal, Y.; Miccoli, P. Bupivacaine 0.5% versus ropivacaine 0.75% wound infiltration to decrease postoperative pain in total thyroidectomy, a prospective controlled study. *Minerva Chir.* **2012**, *67*, 511–516.
12. Li, X.; Yu, L.; Yang, J.; Tan, H. Multimodal analgesia with ropivacaine wound infiltration and intravenous flurbiprofen axetil provides enhanced analgesic effects after radical thyroidectomy: A randomized controlled trial. *BMC Anesthesiol.* **2019**, *19*, 167.
13. Ghlichloo, I.; Gerriets, V. Nonsteroidal Anti-Inflammatory Drugs (NSAIDs) [Updated 2023 May 1]. In *StatPearls*; StatPearls Publishing: Treasure Island, FL, USA, 2023. Available online: https://www.ncbi.nlm.nih.gov/books/NBK547742/ (accessed on 15 May 2024).
14. Benyamin, R.; Trescot, A.M.; Datta, S.; Buenaventura, R.; Adlaka, R.; Sehgal, N.; Glaser, S.E.; Vallejo, R. Opioid complications and side effects. *Pain Physician* **2008**, *11* (Suppl. S2), S105–S120. [CrossRef] [PubMed]
15. Lee, C.; Song, Y.-K.; Jeong, H.-M.; Park, S.-N. The effects of magnesium sulfate infiltration on perioperative opioid consumption and opioid-induced hyperalgesia in patients undergoing robot-assisted laparoscopic prostatectomy with remifentanil-based anesthesia. *Korean J. Anesthesiol.* **2011**, *61*, 244–250. [CrossRef]
16. Razavi, S.S.; Peyvandi, H.; Jam, A.R.B.; Safari, F.; Teymourian, H.; Mohajerani, S.A. Versus Bupivacaine Infiltration in Controlling Postoperative Pain in Inguinal Hernia Repair. *Anesth. Pain Med.* **2015**, *5*, e30643. [CrossRef]
17. Karaaslan, K.; Yilmaz, F.; Gulcu, N.; Sarpkaya, A.; Colak, C.; Kocoglu, H. The effects of levobupivacaine versus levobupivacaine plus magnesium infiltration on postoperative analgesia and laryngospasm in pediatric tonsillectomy patients. *Int. J. Pediatr. Otorhinolaryngol.* **2008**, *72*, 675–681. [CrossRef]
18. Derbel, R.; Achour, I.; Thabet, W.; Chakroun, A.; Zouch, I.; Charfeddine, I. Addition of magnesium sulfate to bupivacaine improves analgesic efficacy after tonsillectomy: A randomized trial and a CONSORT analysis. *Eur. Ann. Otorhinolaryngol. Head Neck. Dis.* **2022**, *139*, 327–331. [CrossRef] [PubMed]
19. Sun, J.; Wu, X.; Zhao, X.; Chen, F.; Wang, W. Pre-emptive peritonsillar infiltration of magnesium sulphate and ropivacaine vs. ropivacaine or magnesium alone for relief of post-adenotonsillectomy pain in children. *Int. J. Pediatr. Otorhinolaryngol.* **2015**, *79*, 499–503. [CrossRef]
20. Sane, S.; Mahdkhah, A.; Golabi, P.; Hesami, S.A.; Kazemi Haki, B. Comparison the effect of bupivacaine plus magnesium sulfate with ropivacaine plus magnesium sulfate infiltration on postoperative pain in patients undergoing lumbar laminectomy with general anesthesia. *Br. J. Neurosurg.* **2020**, *17*, 1–4. [CrossRef] [PubMed]
21. Hazarika, R.; Parua, S.; Choudhury, D.; Barooah, R.K. Comparison of Bupivacaine Plus Magnesium Sulfate and Ropivacaine Plus Magnesium Sulfate Infiltration for Postoperative Analgesia in Patients Undergoing Lumbar Laminectomy: A Randomized Double-blinded Study. *Anesth. Essays Res.* **2017**, *11*, 686–691. [CrossRef] [PubMed] [PubMed Central]
22. Dave, S.; Gopalakrishnan, K.; Krishnan, S.; Natarajan, N. Analgesic Efficacy of Addition of Magnesium Sulfate to Bupivacaine in Wound Infiltration Technique in Perianal Surgeries. *Anesth. Essays Res.* **2022**, *16*, 250–254. [CrossRef] [PubMed] [PubMed Central]
23. Wang, Q.; Zhao, C.; Hu, J.; Ma, T.; Yang, J.; Kang, P. Efficacy of a Modified Cocktail for Periarticular Local Infiltration Analgesia in Total Knee Arthroplasty: A Prospective, Double-Blinded, Randomized Controlled Trial. *J. Bone Jt. Surg.* **2023**, *105*, 354–362. [CrossRef] [PubMed]
24. Zhao, C.; Wang, L.; Chen, L.; Wang, Q.; Kang, P. Effects of magnesium sulfate on periarticular infiltration analgesia in total knee arthroplasty: A prospective, double-blind, randomized controlled trial. *J. Orthop. Surg. Res.* **2023**, *18*, 301. [CrossRef] [PubMed] [PubMed Central]
25. George, A.M.; Liu, M. Ropivacaine. [Updated 2023 Jul 31]. In *StatPearls*; StatPearls Publishing: Treasure Island, FL, USA, 2023. Available online: https://www.ncbi.nlm.nih.gov/books/NBK532924/ (accessed on 16 June 2024).
26. Graf, B.M.; Abraham, I.; Eberbach, N.; Kunst, G.; Stowe, D.F.; Martin, E. Differences in cardiotoxicity of bupivacaine and ropivacaine are the result of physicochemical and stereoselective properties. *Anesthesiology* **2002**, *96*, 1427–1434. [CrossRef]
27. Motamed, C.; Merle, J.C.; Combes, X.; Yahkou, L.; Saidi, N.E.; Degranges, P.; Dhonneur, G. Postthyroidectomy pain control using ropivacaine wound infiltration after intraoperative remifentanil: A prospective double blind randomized controlled study. *Acute Pain.* **2007**, *9*, 119–123. [CrossRef]
28. Karamanlioglu, B.; Turan, A.; Memis, D.; Kaya, G.; Ozata, S.; Ture, M. Infiltration with ropivacaine plus lornoxicam reduces postoperative pain and opioid consumption. *Can. J. Anaesth.* **2005**, *52*, 1047–1053. [CrossRef]

29. Kilbas, Z.; Mentes, M.Ö.; Harlak, A.; Yigit, T.; Balkan, S.M.; Cosar, A.; Öztürk, E.; Kozak, O.; Tufan, C.T. Efficacy of wound infiltration with lornoxicam for postoperative analgesia following thyroidectomy: A prospective, randomized, double-blind study. *Turk. J. Med. Sci.* **2015**, *45*, 700–705. [CrossRef]
30. Yücel, A.; Yazıcı, A.; Müderris, T.; Gül, F. Comparison of lornoxicam and low-dose tramadol for management of post-thyroidectomy pain. *Agriculture* **2016**, *28*, 183–189. [CrossRef] [PubMed]
31. Ledowski, T.; Ang, B.; Schmarbeck, T.; Rhodes, J. Monitoring of sympathetic tone to assess postoperative pain: Skin conductance vs surgical stress index. *Anaesthesia* **2009**, *64*, 727e31. [CrossRef]
32. Jensen, E.W.; Valencia, J.F.; López, A.; Anglada, T.; Agustí, M.; Ramos, Y.; Serra, R.; Jospin, M.; Pineda, P.; Gambus, P. Monitoring hypnotic effect and nociception with two EEG-derived indices, qCON and qNOX, during general anaesthesia. *Acta Anaesthesiol. Scand* **2014**, *58*, 933e41. [CrossRef]
33. Jakuscheit, A.; Weth, J.; Lichtner, G.; Jurth, C.; Rehberg, B.; von Dincklage, F. Intraoperative monitoring of analgesia using nociceptive reflexes correlates with delayed extubation and immediate postoperative pain: A prospective observational study. *Eur. J. Anaesthesiol.* **2017**, *34*, 297e305. [CrossRef] [PubMed]
34. Ledowski, T. Objective monitoring of nociception: A review of current commercial solutions. *Br. J. Anaesth.* **2019**, *123*, e312–e321. [CrossRef] [PubMed] [PubMed Central]
35. Hirose, M.; Okutani, H.; Hashimoto, K.; Ueki, R.; Shimode, N.; Kariya, N.; Takao, Y.; Tatara, T. Intraoperative Assessment of Surgical Stress Response Using Nociception Monitor under General Anesthesia and Postoperative Complications: A Narrative Review. *J. Clin. Med.* **2022**, *11*, 6080. [CrossRef] [PubMed] [PubMed Central]

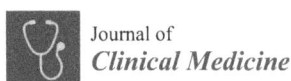

Journal of
Clinical Medicine

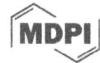

Brief Report

Pain Management and Functional Recovery after Pericapsular Nerve Group (PENG) Block for Total Hip Arthroplasty: A Prospective, Randomized, Double-Blinded Clinical Trial

Małgorzata Domagalska [1,*], Bahadir Ciftci [2], Tomasz Reysner [1], Jerzy Kolasiński [3], Katarzyna Wieczorowska-Tobis [1] and Grzegorz Kowalski [1]

1   Department of Palliative Medicine, University of Medical Sciences, 61-245 Poznan, Poland; tomrey@wp.pl (T.R.); kwt@tobis.pl (K.W.-T.); gkowalski@ump.edu.pl (G.K.)
2   Department of Anesthesiology and Reanimation, Istanbul Medipol University, Istanbul 34214, Turkey; bciftci@medipol.edu.tr
3   Kolasinski Clinic, Hair Clinic Poznan, 62-020 Swarzedz, Poland; colas@klinikakolasinski.pl
*   Correspondence: m.domagalska@icloud.com; Tel./Fax: +48-61-873-83-03

Abstract: Background: The immediate postoperative period after total hip arthroplasty can be associated with significant pain. Therefore, this study aimed to evaluate the effect of pericapsular nerve block on pain management and functional recovery after total hip arthroplasty. Methods: This prospective, randomized, double-blinded, placebo-controlled trial was conducted on 489 adult patients scheduled for total hip arthroplasty, ASA 1–2, operated under spinal analgesia. Participants were assigned to receive either a pericapsular nerve group (PENG) block with 20 mL of 0.5% ropivacaine or a sham block. Results: The primary outcome measure was the postoperative NRS score in motion. The secondary outcomes were cumulative opioid consumption, the time to the first opioid, and functional recovery. Demographic characteristics were similar in both groups. Intraoperative pain scores were significantly lower in patients who received the PENG block than in the control group ($p < 0.0001$). Also, the time to the first opioid was considerably longer in the PENG group ($p < 0.0001$). Additionally, 24% of PENG patients did not require opioids ($p < 0.0001$). Conclusions: The pericapsular nerve group showed significantly decreased opioid consumption and improved functional recovery. Pericapsular nerve group block improved pain management and postoperative functional recovery following total hip arthroplasty.

Keywords: total hip arthroplasty; PENG block; quality of life; pain management; regional anesthesia

Citation: Domagalska, M.; Ciftci, B.; Reysner, T.; Kolasiński, J.; Wieczorowska-Tobis, K.; Kowalski, G. Pain Management and Functional Recovery after Pericapsular Nerve Group (PENG) Block for Total Hip Arthroplasty: A Prospective, Randomized, Double-Blinded Clinical Trial. *J. Clin. Med.* **2023**, *12*, 4931. https://doi.org/10.3390/jcm12154931

Academic Editors: Felice Eugenio Agro, Giuseppe Pascarella and Fabio Costa

Received: 8 June 2023
Revised: 15 July 2023
Accepted: 18 July 2023
Published: 27 July 2023

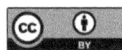
1. Introduction

Total hip arthroplasty is one of the most common major orthopedic interventions and improves patients' quality of life and functional status [1]. However, despite these advantages, the immediate time after surgery can be associated with significant pain, which delays mobilization and increases the duration of hospitalization and the risk of thromboembolic events [2,3]. In total hip arthroplasty (THR), the pain is usually treated with an injection of a local anesthetic around the joint, known as "local infiltration analgesia". Adequate pain management after total hip arthroplasty is critical for early rehabilitation and patient satisfaction. Moreover, the complex innervation of the hip joint makes a perfect regional anesthesia technique questionable. After surgery, regional anesthesia techniques for pain management include epidural analgesia, lumbar plexus block, parasacral block, fascia iliaca block, and femoral and obturator nerve block [2,4,5]. However, these procedures can lead to complications such as epidural hematoma, headache after surgery, or prolonged motor block with the subsequent prolonged hospital stay [6–8].

The obturator nerves, accessory obturator, and femoral nerve innervate the anterior hip capsule. The iliopubic eminence and inferomedial acetabulum were recommended as important bone landmarks to block the articular branches of these three nerves. Furthermore, the great role of the accessory obturator nerve and femoral nerve in the anterior hip innervation has also been stated.

LIA pursues the sensory nerve endings around the joints without decreasing the quadriceps strength. However, even with LIA, some patients experience pain in the days after total hip arthroplasty.

An international consensus of evidence-based experts recommends peripheral nerve blocks (PNB) as a central anesthetic method in THA to improve outcomes [9]. PNB for postoperative analgesia would also maintain quadriceps strength to facilitate early recovery. Common PNBs like a sciatic nerve block, femoral nerve block, lumbar plexus block, and fascia iliaca block cause quadriceps muscle weakness.

The pericapsular nerve group (PENG) block is an ultrasound-guided approach first described by Giron-Arango et al. [10]. The PENG block targets the articular branches of the obturator nerve, the accessory obturator nerve, and the femoral nerve, providing sensory innervation to the anterior capsule of the hip [7,11,12]. It has been used successfully in multimodal pain management for hip fractures [12,13] and for pain management after total hip arthroplasty [14]. It has been shown that the PENG block can protect the body, speeding up the first ambulance and recovery. However, some studies have shown that it can weaken the quadriceps, especially if the volume is more than 20 mL [15,16]. Therefore, we conducted a prospective, randomized, controlled, double-blinded trial to assess the effectiveness of a PENG block in improving analgesia and functional recovery following total hip arthroplasty. Our primary outcomes were the postoperative pain sores, and the secondary outcome measures included opioid consumption and functional recovery expressed by active elevation of the operated limb and walking by the balcony.

2. Patients and Methods

2.1. Study Design and Participants

This prospective, randomized trial was performed at the Independent Public Health Care Institution of the Ministry of the Interior and Administration in Poznań, Poland, in accordance with the Declaration of Helsinki. The Institutional Review Board of the Poznan University of Medical Sciences approved the study protocol on 17 June 2020, protocol number 496/20, and registered it at clinicaltrails.gov (NCT05944380). Written informed consent was obtained from all patients for this scientific contribution.

Enrollment was proposed before surgery for adults scheduled for elective primary unilateral total hip arthroplasty under spinal anesthesia, aged >18 years, and American Society of Anesthesiologists physical status 1 or 2.

Patients were not included in this study if they refused to participate, had a history of opioid abuse, had an infection of the site of needle puncture, were less than 18 years of age, were postponed as having ASA > 2, had an allergy to any of the drugs used in the study, had renal failure (estimated glomerular filtration rate of <15 mL/min/1.73 m^2), liver failure, known or suspected coagulopathy, pre-existing anatomical or neurological disorders in the lower extremities, intellectual disability with problems in pain evaluation, and severe psychiatric illness.

2.2. Randomization

Patients were randomly allocated to receive ultrasound-guided PENG block, or sham block, by computer software using a 1:1 randomization list generated by the program nQuery Advisor (Statistical Solutions, Boston, MA, USA). The randomization lists were accessible to a researcher who was not involved in the study and concealed group assignments in consecutively numbered, sealed, opaque envelopes. A consultant anesthesiologist followed management to open the envelopes shortly before the nerve block performance to reveal the group allocation and perform the procedure according to the assignment. The patients, surgeons, operating room staff, and anesthesia team were masked from the study group allocation. Group blinding and unmasking occurred once the statistical analysis was complete.

All patients underwent primary total hip replacement (under spinal analgesia) performed by three surgical teams using the posterior approach at our tertiary institution.

The study subjects were subjected to at least 5 days of active follow-up. An independent researcher gathered the primary and secondary outcomes during in-person hospital visits.

2.3. Perioperative Management and Spinal Anesthesia Procedure

All the patients received standardized spinal anesthetic management as commonly practiced in our hospital. In both groups, the patients received 7.5 mg of midazolam p.o. and 8 mg of Dexamethasone i.v. half an hour before the procedure as a part of multimodal preemptive analgesia. For mild sedation, before the induction of anesthesia, intravenous doses of 2 mg of midazolam and 100 mg of fentanyl were given. In addition, all patients had spinal anesthesia, which was performed by injecting 20 mg of ropivacaine 0.5% through a 27G or 25G Whitacre needle at the L2–L3 or L3–L4 interspace with the patient sitting. Intravenous tranexamic acid 1000 mg and cefazolin 1 g were administered after spinal anesthesia and before surgery. There was no surgeon-delivered periarticular infiltration during the surgery.

2.4. PENG Block Procedure

In both groups, the PENG block or sham block was performed after the spinal anesthesia and before the surgical incision, according to the technique described by Girón-Arango [10]. However, according to Peng et al. [17] and Tran et al. [18], we modified the original PENG block technique to avoid quadriceps weakness. A curvilinear probe (low frequency, 4–8 mHz) was used. The puncture was performed in the lateromedial direction, and the needle was placed more laterally, away from the surface of the iliopsoas tendon and between the anteroinferior iliac spine and the ilio-pubic eminence. After negative aspiration, 20 mL of 0.5% ropivacaine or 20 mL of 0.9% NaCl was injected laterally from the iliopsoas tendon, as seen in Figure 1. Three anesthesiologists performed the blocks. All had at least five years of experience of post-specialty clinical experience focused on regional anesthesia. During the surgery, basic hemodynamic parameters, opioid consumption (fentanyl), and operation time were measured.

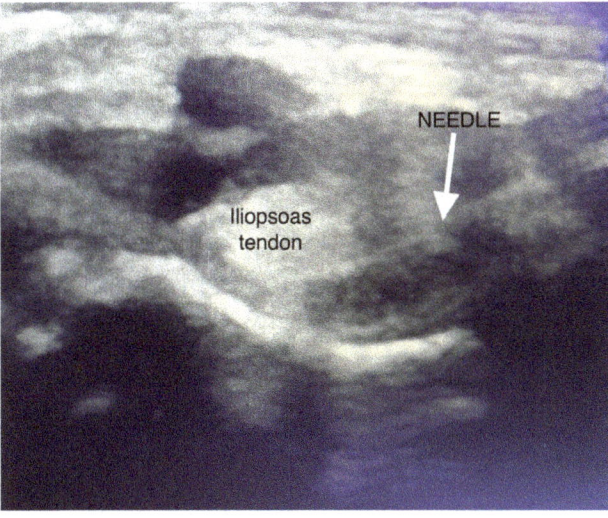

Figure 1. Injection technique of PENG block.

2.5. Postoperative Analgesia Management and Evaluation of Outcomes

The patients were transferred to the post-anesthesia care unit (PACU) after the end of the surgery. In the PACU, the same postoperative multimodal analgesia was applied in both groups, which was consistent with acetaminophen 1 g i.v. every six hours, metamizole 1 g i.v. every six hours, and ketorolac 50 mg every twelve hours. The 5 mg morphine was administered if the NRS score was higher than 4 as rescue analgesia. When severe nausea or vomiting occurred, the patients were treated with 8 mg of Ondansentrone. All patients received thromboembolism prophylaxis daily with enoxaparin for 4 weeks postoperatively. Subsequently, after the first 10 postoperative hours, patients were ambulated with the help of the hiker.

2.6. Outcome Assessments

The primary outcome measures were pain scores at rest and during mobilization up to 5 days following surgery. At all postoperative time points (24, 48, 72, >72 h), patients were asked to rate perceived pain using an 11-point Numeric Pain Rating Scale (NRS: 0 indicating no pain and 10 indicating the worst pain imaginable) experienced at rest and during mobilization. The secondary outcomes included total opioid consumption and time to first opioid use obtained from the postoperative and orthopedic wards. Opioid consumption during 0–24, 24–48, and 48–72 h after surgery, and total opioid consumption at 72 h following surgery, were recorded. The consumption of the different types of postoperative opioid administration was converted to intravenous morphine equivalents. The functional recovery of each patient was tested by active elevation of the operated limb. The measurement was made 6 h postoperatively, and the ability to walk 3 steps by the balcony was assessed 10 h after surgery.

The outcome assessment was performed by a group of two clinicians (GK and KWT) who were blinded to the group allocation.

2.7. Statistical Analyses and Sample Size Calculation

To calculate the sample size, we studied our primary and secondary hypotheses that the PENG block improves postoperative analgesia. We estimated pain score density as a mean of 4 and SD of 6 based on the published data on total hip arthroplasty using PENG blocks [14]. We use a truncated Gaussian distribution with a range of 0 to 10, SD 6, and a mean of 4 for the PENG group to model the drift. Under these assumptions and two-sided = 5%, we simulated a sample of 234 patients in each group. With an overall sample size of 468 subjects, we estimated 95% power to detect differences in pain between groups as small as approximately 1. Statistical analysis was performed using GraphPad Prism 8 software (GraphPad Software Inc., San Diego, CA, USA).

The parametric distribution of numerical variables was evaluated using the Kołomogorov–Smirnov normality test. The differences between groups were analyzed by t-student or Mann–Whitney U test. Categorical variables were correlated with the Mann–Whitney U test, and an analysis of contingency was compared with Fisher's exact test. Values are given as mean (standard deviation), median (interquartile range), or the number of patients (proportion). The balance of inpatient and operation idiosyncrasies between the randomized groups was determined by estimating the standardized difference, defined as the variation in proportions or means divided by the pooled standard deviation. Successively measured variables were postponed using a linear mixed model with the patient indicator as a random effect and group, time, and group-by-time interaction as fixed effects, adjusting for variables of patient and operation characteristics (sex, age, body mass index, ASA physical status, surgery duration, spinal anesthesia level). An unstructured covariance structure was applied. The Bonferroni correction was enforced to adapt for multiple comparisons. All analyses were accomplished using GraphPad Prism 8 software (GraphPad Software Inc., San Diego, CA, USA). A *p*-value of <0.05 was treated as statistically significant.

3. Results

Patients and Operation Characteristics

Of 556 patients assessed for eligibility, 43 did not meet the inclusion criteria, and 24 preferred general anesthesia. The remaining 489 were randomly allocated between groups, as shown in Figure 2. No clinically relevant differences were apparent from group characteristics, as shown in Table 1.

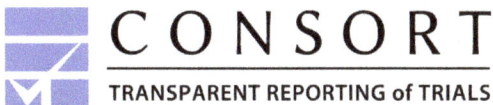

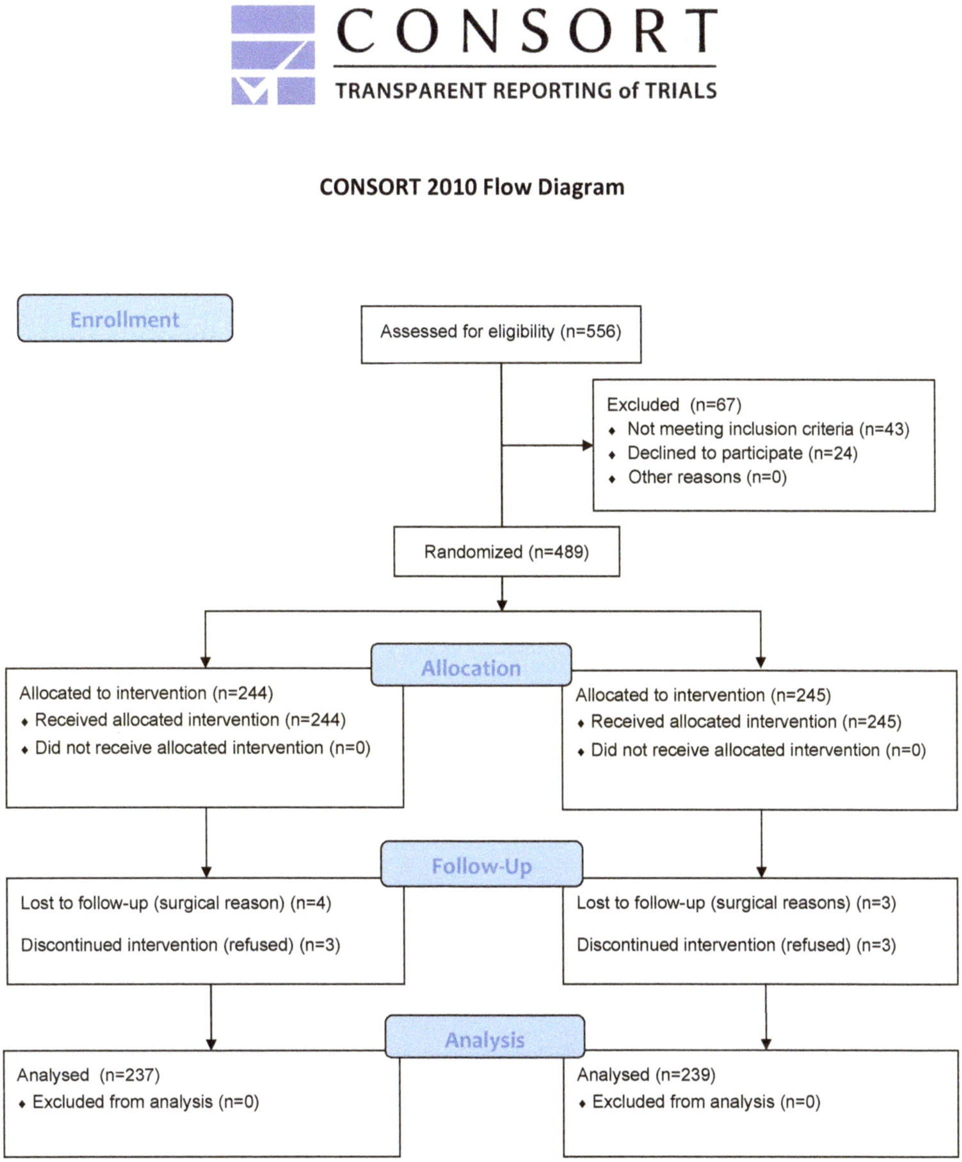
CONSORT
TRANSPARENT REPORTING of TRIALS
CONSORT 2010 Flow Diagram
Enrollment
Assessed for eligibility (n=556)
Excluded (n=67)
• Not meeting inclusion criteria (n=43)
• Declined to participate (n=24)
• Other reasons (n=0)
Randomized (n=489)
Allocation
Allocated to intervention (n=244)
• Received allocated intervention (n=244)
• Did not receive allocated intervention (n=0)
Allocated to intervention (n=245)
• Received allocated intervention (n=245)
• Did not receive allocated intervention (n=0)
Follow-Up
Lost to follow-up (surgical reason) (n=4)
Discontinued intervention (refused) (n=3)
Lost to follow-up (surgical reasons) (n=3)
Discontinued intervention (refused) (n=3)
Analysis
Analysed (n=237)
• Excluded from analysis (n=0)
Analysed (n=239)
• Excluded from analysis (n=0)

Figure 2. Consort Flow Chart.

Table 1. Baseline characteristics. Values are mean (SD) or number.

	Sham Block Group n = 237	Pericapsular Nerve Group (PENG) Block Group n = 239	*p* Value
ASA	2 (SD = 0.5)	2 (SD = 0.5)	0.8508
Age (years)	66 (SD = 5.1)	66 (SD = 5.8)	0.1001
Sex (F/M)	115/122	99/140	0.1429
BMI (kg/m^2)	31 (SD = 2.9)	31 (SD = 3.2)	0.2108
NRS at rest—before surgery	4.1 (SD = 1.3)	4.3 (SD = 1.1)	0.2741
Spinal anesthesia needle level (L2/3 vs. L3/4)	31 (13%) vs. 206 (87%)	34 (14%) vs. 205 (86%)	0.7898
Surgery duration (min)	63 (SD = 7.6)	61 (SD = 8.3)	0.3211

ASA—American Society of Anesthesiologists Physical Status Classification System; F—female; M—male; BMI—body mass index; PENG—pericapsular nerve group.

Postoperative pain scores are shown in Table 2 and Figures 2 and 3. Patients who underwent the PENG block had lower NRS pain scores at rest at all time points. Comparing the PENG block to the sham block, NRS pain scores such as 3.1 vs. 5.3 at 24 h ($p < 0.0001$), 2.8 vs. 2.5 at 72 h ($p < 0.0001$), and 0.4 vs. 0 over 72 h ($p = 0.0004$), reveals better pain control.

Table 2. Study outcomes. Values are mean (SD) or numbers.

	Sham Block Group n = 237	Pericapsular Nerve Group (PENG) Block Group n = 239	*p* Value
NRS postoperative			
24 h	5.3 (SD = 1.0)	3.1 (SD = 1.0)	<0.0001
NRS in motion			
48 h	7.6 (SD = 1.0)	5.9 (SD = 1.0)	<0.0001
72 h	6.4 (SD = 1.1)	5.2 (SD = 0.6)	<0.0001
>72 h	5.7 (SD = 1.0)	4.4 (SD = 0.6)	<0.0001
NRS at rest			
48 h	3.7 (SD = 0.7)	2.8 (SD = 0.8)	<0.0001
72 h	2.8 (SD = 0.6)	2.5 (SD = 0.8)	<0.0001
>72 h	0.4 (SD = 0.8)	0	0.0004
Postoperative opioid consumption			
yes	237 (100%)	182 (76%)	<0.0001
no	0 (0%)	57 (24%)	
Time to first opioid			
hours	4.5 (SD = 1.6)	9.5 (SD = 5.5)	<0.0001
Total opioid consumption(Intravenous morphine equivalents; mg)			
0–24 h	8.4 (SD = 3.7)	2.3 (SD = 1.6)	<0.0001
24–48 h	2.5 (SD = 2.0)	0.5 (SD = 1.1)	<0.0001
48–72 h	0.3 (SD = 0.7)	0	<0.0001
Functional recovery			
Active elevation of operated limb	25 (11%)	127 (53%)	<0.0001
Walking by the balcony	108 (46%)	239 (100%)	<0.0001

NRS, numerical rating scale; mg, milligrams.

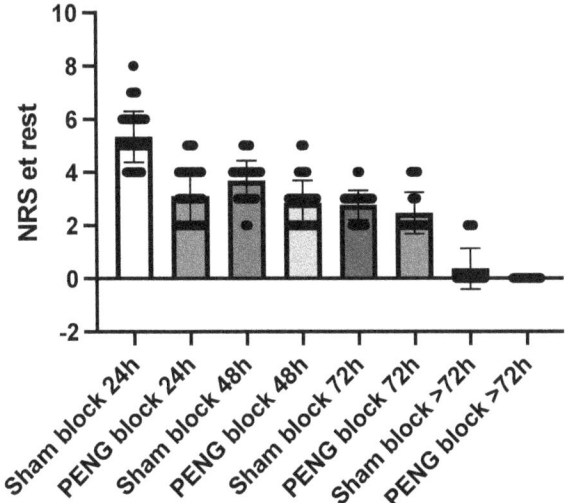

Figure 3. NRS at rest.

Also, NRS pain scores during movement were lower in the PENG block group at all time points, with a median of 5.9 vs. 7.6 at 48 h, 5.2 vs. 6.4 at 72 h, and 4.4 vs. 5.7 over 72 h, all $p < 0.0001$ (Figure 4).

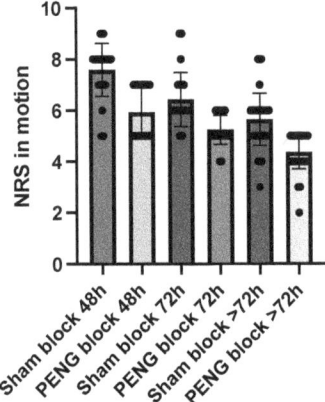

Figure 4. NRS et motion.

Every patient in the Sham group received morphine intravenously for pain treatment. In contrast, 57 (24%) in the PENG group received none. As a result, the total opioid consumption, expressed in intravenous equivalents, was lower in the PENG group at all time points: 2.3 vs. 8.4 at 24 h, 0.5 vs. 2.5 at 48 h, and 0 vs. 0.3 at 72 h, all $p < 0.0001$. In addition, the mean time to the first opioid was 5 h shorter in the Sham group ($p < 0.0001$) (Figure 5). The results are shown in Table 2.

Quadriceps Strength in the operative leg measured 6 h after surgery by active elevation of the operated limb was higher in the PENG group. 127 (53%) patients in the PENG group could actively elevate the operated limb, compared to 25 (11%) patients in the Sham group. The remaining 47% of patients in the PENG group and 75% of patients in the Sham group could not actively elevate the operated limb due to accompanying pain.

Time to first opioid

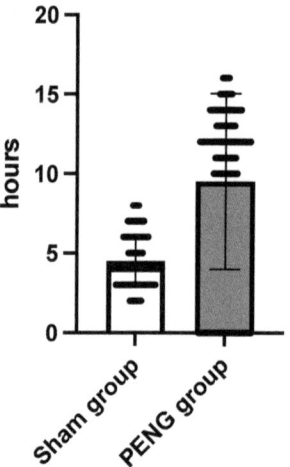

Figure 5. Time to first opioid.

Moreover, all patients in the PENG group could walk by the balcony 10 h after surgery, compared to 108 (47%) in the sham group, $p < 0.0001$. 53% of patients in the Sham group could not walk by the balcony due to accompanying pain.

4. Discussion

The major result of this study was that ultrasound-guided PENG block could improve pain relief after surgery in THA patients without weakening the quadriceps muscle. Additionally, patients in the PENG group took much longer until the first opioid, and half did not require opioids. Our results support the fact that the pericapsular nerve group significantly reduced pain scores during motion and opioid consumption. Moreover, it extended the time until the first opioid and improved functional recovery.

The PENG block is a relatively novel ultrasound-guided regional anesthesia technique designed to block the branches of the femoral, obturator, and obturator accessory nerves innervating the anterior capsule of the hip joint [10,14]. Currently, the PENG block is used for pain management in various hip surgeries, including fractures and hip replacements [11–14,17]. However, most recent evidence is limited to trials with small group sizes [11,14] and case reports [19–22]. Pascarella et al. [14], in their randomized, observer-masked, controlled trial, showed a significant reduction in opioid consumption, a shorter time to ambulation, and a better range of hip motion. Also, Lin et al. [16], in their double-blinded randomized comparative trial, showed that patients receiving PENG block for intraoperative and postoperative analgesia during hip fracture surgery experienced less postoperative pain with preserved quadriceps strength. Similar pain relief was also observed in our study. On the other hand, Zheng et al. [23] revealed that a PENG block added to intra-articular injection of local anesthetic provides a limited benefit to postoperative analgesia. However, Eti Korkusuz et al. [24] showed that ultrasound-guided PENG block offers better pain relief in treating hip osteoarthritis than the intra-articular injection of steroid-bupivacaine.

Quadriceps weakness was observed in some studies after the PENG block [16,25,26]. The exact mechanism of femoral nerve anesthesia after PENG block is controversial and results from local anesthetic spread via a plane between the psoas major and pectineus or intramuscularly [27]. According to Pascarella et al. [28] to avoid the short-term motor block, the needle tip should be placed medial to the iliopsoas eminence and under the iliopsoas tendon. Also, the clinician should observe a transversal spread with the tendon lifted during the injection. In our study, we placed the needle tip laterally and away from the undersurface of the iliopsoas tendon. Also, we reduced the volume of a local anesthetic to 20 mL to avoid motor weakness, as Çiftçi et al. [29] and Yeoh et al. [30] suggested in their studies. For this reason, we did not observe quadriceps weakness in our study. However, in our study, 47% of patients in the PENG group and 75% in the Sham group could not actively elevate the operated limb. The severe pain caused difficulty lifting the operated limb, similar to other studies [31,32].

A significant drawback of a single-shot PENG block is the limited time of analgesia. Also, rebound hyperalgesia after a single-shot nerve block has been reported [33,34]. Therefore, our study gave the patients acetaminophen, metamizole, and ketorolac to avoid rebound pain. Also, we decided to use systematic dexamethasone to prolong analgesia following a single-shot peripheral nerve block due to its proven effectiveness [35].

Only three researchers [10,19,36] reported that few patients experienced pain after the PENG block in the lateral femoral cutaneous nerve region. That is why we decided not to add the femoral cutaneous nerve block to the PENG block. In addition, we did not observe pain in the femoral cutaneous nerve region in our study. Furthermore, the pain scores were significantly lower in the PENG group, and 24% of patients did not need opioids, compared to 0% in the placebo group. Furthermore, the PENG block significantly reduced total opioid consumption and lengthened the time to first opioid consumption. Also, total opioid consumption was lower in the PENG group, and the patients in the PENG group did not require opioids 48 h postoperatively.

Our study suggests that the PENG block maintained optimal postoperative pain management, swift motor recovery, and lowered opioid consumption. Therefore, the PENG block may be a helpful anesthetic technique for postoperative pain control in modern, rapid hip surgery.

However, this study has limitations, such as the volume of the local anesthetic used for the PENG block, single-shot injection instead of the catheter, and the fact that we did not evaluate the dermatome levels. The functional recovery was assessed by active elevation of the operated limb 6 h after surgery and the ability to walk 3 steps by the balcony 10 h after surgery. Our study included only posterior total hip replacements, although this is the most commonly performed procedure worldwide.

5. Conclusions

The PENG block has proven to be a forceful opioid-sparing analgesic technique that boosts early postoperative mobilization and merits consideration as an effective analgesic option in total hip arthroplasty.

Author Contributions: All of the authors (M.D., B.C., T.R., K.W.-T., J.K. and G.K.) made substantial contributions to the conception and design, or acquisition of data, or analysis and interpretation of data; they have been involved in drafting the manuscript or revising it critically for important intellectual content; have given final approval of the version to be published. All authors have read and agreed to the published version of the manuscript.

Funding: This research received no external funding.

Institutional Review Board Statement: The study was conducted in accordance with the Declaration of Helsinki, and approved by the Institutional Review Board of Poznan University of Medical Science on 17 June 2020, protocol number 496/20.

Informed Consent Statement: Informed consent was obtained from all subjects involved in the study.

Data Availability Statement: The study datasets are available from the corresponding author at reasonable request.

Conflicts of Interest: The authors declare that they have no known competing financial interest or personal relationships that could have appeared to influence the work reported in this paper.

References

1. Fontalis, A.; Epinette, J.-A.; Thaler, M.; Zagra, L.; Khanduja, V.; Haddad, F.S. Advances and innovations in total hip arthroplasty. *SICOT-J* **2021**, *7*, 26. [CrossRef] [PubMed]
2. Surace, P.; Sultan, A.A.; George, J.; Samuel, L.T.; Khlopas, A.; Molloy, R.M.; Stearns, K.L.; Mont, M.A. The association between operative time and short-term complications in total hip arthroplasty: An analysis of 89,802 surgeries. *J. Arthroplast.* **2019**, *34*, 426–432. [CrossRef] [PubMed]
3. Wu, V.J.; Ross, B.J.; Sanchez, F.L.; Billings, C.R.; Sherman, W.F. Complications following total hip arthroplasty: A nationwide database study comparing elective vs hip fracture cases. *J. Arthroplast.* **2020**, *35*, 2144–2148. [CrossRef] [PubMed]
4. Zhao, J.; Davis, S.P. An integrative review of multimodal pain management on patient recovery after total hip and knee arthroplasty. *Int. J. Nurs. Stud.* **2019**, *98*, 94–106. [CrossRef]
5. Laigaard, J.; Pedersen, C.; Rønsbo, T.N.; Mathiesen, O.; Karlsen, A.P.H. Minimal clinically important differences in randomised clinical trials on pain management after total hip and knee arthroplasty: A systematic review. *Br. J. Anaesth.* **2021**, *126*, 1029–1037. [CrossRef]
6. Marty, P.; Chassery, C.; Rontes, O.; Vuillaume, C.; Basset, B.; Merouani, M.; Marquis, C.; De Lussy, A.; Ferré, F.; Naudin, C. Combined proximal or distal nerve blocks for postoperative analgesia after total knee arthroplasty: A randomised controlled trial. *Br. J. Anaesth.* **2022**, *129*, 427–434. [CrossRef]
7. Sousa, I.P.; da Silva Peixoto, C.L.; Coimbra, L.F.; da Costa Rodrigues, F. Comparison of pericapsular nerve group (PENG) block and epidural analgesia following total hip arthroplasty: A retrospective analysis. *Rev. Española Anestesiol. Y Reanim.* **2022**, *69*, 632–639. [CrossRef]
8. Angers, M.; Belzile, É.L.; Vachon, J.; Beauchamp-Chalifour, P.; Pelet, S. Negative influence of femoral nerve block on quadriceps strength recovery following total knee replacement: A prospective randomized trial. *Orthop. Traumatol. Surg. Res.* **2019**, *105*, 633–637. [CrossRef]
9. Memtsoudis, S.G.; Cozowicz, C.; Bekeris, J.; Bekere, D.; Liu, J.; Soffin, E.M.; Mariano, E.R.; Johnson, R.L.; Go, G.; Hargett, M.J. Peripheral nerve block anesthesia/analgesia for patients undergoing primary hip and knee arthroplasty: Recommendations from the International Consensus on Anesthesia-Related Outcomes after Surgery (ICAROS) group based on a systematic review and meta-analysis of current literature. *Reg. Anesth. Pain Med.* **2021**, *46*, 971–985.
10. Girón-Arango, L.; Peng, P.W.; Chin, K.J.; Brull, R.; Perlas, A. Pericapsular nerve group (PENG) block for hip fracture. *Reg. Anesth. Pain Med.* **2018**, *43*, 859–863. [CrossRef] [PubMed]
11. Aliste, J.; Layera, S.; Bravo, D.; Jara, Á.; Muñoz, G.; Barrientos, C.; Wulf, R.; Brañez, J.; Finlayson, R.J.; Tran, D.Q. Randomized comparison between pericapsular nerve group (PENG) block and suprainguinal fascia iliaca block for total hip arthroplasty. *Reg. Anesth. Pain Med.* **2021**, *46*, 874–878. [CrossRef] [PubMed]
12. Allard, C.; Pardo, E.; de la Jonquière, C.; Wyniecki, A.; Soulier, A.; Faddoul, A.; Tsai, E.S.; Bonnet, F.; Verdonk, F. Comparison between femoral block and PENG block in femoral neck fractures: A cohort study. *PLoS ONE* **2021**, *16*, e0252716. [CrossRef]
13. Hua, H.; Xu, Y.; Jiang, M.; Dai, X. Evaluation of pericapsular nerve group (PENG) block for analgesic effect in elderly patients with femoral neck fracture undergoing hip arthroplasty. *J. Healthc. Eng.* **2022**, *2022*, 7452716. [CrossRef]
14. Pascarella, G.; Costa, F.; Del Buono, R.; Pulitanò, R.; Strumia, A.; Piliego, C.; De Quattro, E.; Cataldo, R.; Agrò, F.; Carassiti, M. Impact of the pericapsular nerve group (PENG) block on postoperative analgesia and functional recovery following total hip arthroplasty: A randomised, observer-masked, controlled trial. *Anaesthesia* **2021**, *76*, 1492–1498. [CrossRef] [PubMed]
15. Bilal, B.; Öksüz, G.; Boran, Ö.F.; Topak, D.; Doğar, F. High volume pericapsular nerve group (PENG) block for acetabular fracture surgery: A new horizon for novel block. *J. Clin. Anesth.* **2020**, *62*, 109702. [CrossRef] [PubMed]
16. Lin, D.-Y.; Morrison, C.; Brown, B.; Saies, A.A.; Pawar, R.; Vermeulen, M.; Anderson, S.R.; Lee, T.S.; Doornberg, J.; Kroon, H.M. Pericapsular nerve group (PENG) block provides improved short-term analgesia compared with the femoral nerve block in hip fracture surgery: A single-center double-blinded randomized comparative trial. *Reg. Anesth. Pain Med.* **2021**, *46*, 398–403. [CrossRef]
17. Peng, P.W.; Perlas, A.; Chin, K.J. Reply to Dr Nielsen: Pericapsular nerve group (PENG) block for hip fracture. *Reg. Anesth. Pain Med.* **2019**, *44*, 415–416. [CrossRef]
18. Tran, J.; Agur, A.; Peng, P. Is pericapsular nerve group (PENG) block a true pericapsular block? *Reg. Anesth. Pain Med.* **2019**, *44*, 257. [CrossRef]
19. Thallaj, A. Combined PENG and LFCN blocks for postoperative analgesia in hip surgery—A case report. *Saudi J. Anaesth.* **2019**, *13*, 381.
20. Pagano, T.; Scarpato, F.; Chicone, G.; Carbone, D.; Bussemi, C.B.; Albano, F.; Ruotolo, F. Analgesic evaluation of ultrasound-guided Pericapsular Nerve Group (PENG) block for emergency hip surgery in fragile patients: A case series. *Arthroplasty* **2019**, *1*, 18. [CrossRef]
21. Kukreja, P.; Schuster, B.; Northern, T.; Sipe, S.; Naranje, S.; Kalagara, H. Pericapsular nerve group (PENG) block in combination with the quadratus lumborum block analgesia for revision total hip arthroplasty: A retrospective case series. *Cureus* **2020**, *12*, e12233. [CrossRef] [PubMed]
22. Singh, S.; Ahmed, W. Continuous pericapsular nerve group block for hip surgery: A case series. *A&A Pract.* **2020**, *14*, e01320.
23. Zheng, J.; Pan, D.; Zheng, B.; Ruan, X. Preoperative pericapsular nerve group (PENG) block for total hip arthroplasty: A randomized, placebo-controlled trial. *Reg. Anesth. Pain Med.* **2022**, *47*, 155–160. [PubMed]

24. Et, T.; Korkusuz, M. Comparison of pericapsular nerve group (peng) block with intra-articular and quadratus lumborum block in primary total hip arthroplasty: A randomized controlled trial. *Korean J. Anesthesiol.* **2023**. *ahead of print*. [CrossRef] [PubMed]
25. Choi, Y.S.; Park, K.K.; Lee, B.; Nam, W.S.; Kim, D.-H. Pericapsular Nerve Group (PENG) block versus supra-inguinal fascia iliaca compartment block for total hip arthroplasty: A randomized clinical trial. *J. Pers. Med.* **2022**, *12*, 408. [CrossRef]
26. Senthil, K.; Kumar, P.; Ramakrishnan, L. Comparison of pericapsular nerve group block versus fascia iliaca compartment block as postoperative pain management in hip fracture surgeries. *Anesth. Essays Res.* **2021**, *15*, 352.
27. Yu, H.C.; Moser, J.J.; Chu, A.Y.; Montgomery, S.H.; Brown, N.; Endersby, R.V.W. Inadvertent quadriceps weakness following the pericapsular nerve group (PENG) block. *Reg. Anesth. Pain Med.* **2019**. [CrossRef]
28. Pascarella, G.; Costa, F.; Del Buono, R.; Strumia, A.; Cataldo, R.; Felice, E.A.; Carassiti, M. Defining the optimal spread of local anesthetic during pericapsular nerve group (PENG) block may help to avoid short-term motor block (reply to Aliste et al.). *Reg. Anesth. Pain Med.* **2022**, *47*, 200–201. [CrossRef]
29. Çiftçi, B.; Ahıskalıoğlu, A.; Altıntaş, H.M.; Tekin, B.; Şakul, B.U.; Alıcı, H.A. A possible mechanism of motor blockade of high volume pericapsular nerve group (PENG) block: A cadaveric study. *J. Clin. Anesth.* **2021**, *74*, 110407. [CrossRef]
30. Yeoh, S.-R.; Chou, Y.; Chan, S.-M.; Hou, J.-D.; Lin, J.-A. Pericapsular nerve group block and iliopsoas plane block: A scoping review of quadriceps weakness after two proclaimed motor-sparing Hip blocks. *Healthcare* **2022**, *10*, 1565.
31. Hu, J.; Wang, Q.; Hu, J.; Kang, P.; Yang, J. Efficacy of ultrasound-guided pericapsular nerve group (PENG) block combined with local infiltration analgesia on postoperative pain after total hip arthroplasty: A prospective, double-blind, randomized controlled trial. *J. Arthroplast.* **2023**, *38*, 1096–1103. [CrossRef]
32. Bravo, D.; Aliste, J.; Layera, S.; Fernández, D.; Erpel, H.; Aguilera, G.; Arancibia, H.; Barrientos, C.; Wulf, R.; León, S. Randomized clinical trial comparing pericapsular nerve group (PENG) block and periarticular local anesthetic infiltration for total hip arthroplasty. *Reg. Anesth. Pain Med.* **2023**. [CrossRef] [PubMed]
33. Nobre, L.V.; Cunha, G.P.; Sousa, P.C.C.B.D.; Takeda, A.; Ferraro, L.H.C. Peripheral nerve block and rebound pain: Literature review. *Rev. Bras. Anestesiol.* **2020**, *69*, 587–593. [CrossRef] [PubMed]
34. Dada, O.; Gonzalez Zacarias, A.; Ongaigui, C.; Echeverria-Villalobos, M.; Kushelev, M.; Bergese, S.D.; Moran, K. Does rebound pain after peripheral nerve block for orthopedic surgery impact postoperative analgesia and opioid consumption? A narrative review. *Int. J. Environ. Res. Public Health* **2019**, *16*, 3257.
35. Baeriswyl, M.; Kirkham, K.; Jacot-Guillarmod, A.; Albrecht, E. Efficacy of perineural vs systemic dexamethasone to prolong analgesia after peripheral nerve block: A systematic review and meta-analysis. *BJA Br. J. Anaesth.* **2017**, *119*, 183–191. [CrossRef] [PubMed]
36. Talawar, P.; Tandon, S.; Tripathy, D.; Kaushal, A. Combined pericapsular nerve group and lateral femoral cutaneous nerve blocks for surgical anaesthesia in hip arthroscopy. *Indian J. Anaesth.* **2020**, *64*, 638. [CrossRef]

MDPI AG
Grosspeteranlage 5
4052 Basel
Switzerland
Tel.: +41 61 683 77 34

Journal of Clinical Medicine Editorial Office
E-mail: jcm@mdpi.com
www.mdpi.com/journal/jcm

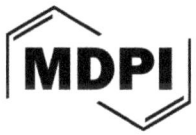

www.ingramcontent.com/pod-product-compliance
Lightning Source LLC
LaVergne TN
LVHW070557100526

838202LV00012B/490